# The Science
## of
# Marijuana

# The
# *Science*
# *of*
# *Marijuana*

*Second Edition*

## Leslie L. Iversen

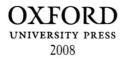

OXFORD
UNIVERSITY PRESS
2008

# OXFORD
UNIVERSITY PRESS

Oxford University Press, Inc., publishes works that further
Oxford University's objective of excellence
in research, scholarship, and education.

Oxford   New York
Auckland   Cape Town   Dares Salaam   Hong Kong   Karachi
Kuala   Lumpur   Madrid   Melbourne   Mexico City   Nairobi
New Delhi   Shanghai   Taipei   Toronto

With offices in
Argentina   Austria   Brazil   Chile   Czech Republic   France   Greece
Guatemala   Hungary   Italy   Japan   Poland   Portugal   Singapore
South Korea   Switzerland   Thailand   Turkey   Ukraine   Vietnam

Published by Oxford University Press, Inc.
198 Madison Avenue, New York, New York 10016
www.oup.com

Oxford is a registered trademark of Oxford University Press

Library of Congress Cataloging-in-Publication Data

Iversen, Leslie L.
The science of marijuana / Leslie L. Iversen—2nd ed.
p.; cm.
ISBN 978-0-19-532824-0
1. Marijuana—Physiological effect. 2. Marijuana—Toxicology.
[DNLM: 1. Tetrahydocannabinol—pharmacology. 2. Cannabis—adverse effects.
3. Central Nervous System—drug effects. 4. Endocannabinoids—physiology.
5. Marijuana Smoking—epidemiology. 6. Tetrahydrocannabinol—therapeutic use.
QV 77.7 I94s 2008] I. Title.
QP801.C27I94 2008
615'.7827—dc22        2007021605

Printed in the United States of America
on acid-free paper

# Foreword

## By Solomon H. Snyder

The history of marijuana is one of déjà vu. One of the oldest drugs in clinical medicine, marijuana extracts were widely used in India and countries of the Far East for thousands of years as sleeping aids, apoptotic stimulants, anti-convulsants, anti-anxiety, and antidepressant medications. In the nineteenth century, the British imported these therapeutic strategies from their Indian colonies, and soon thereafter cannabis was employed extensively in the United States for medical purposes. Recreational use of marijuana expanded in the early twentieth century, leading to draconian suppression in the late 1930s, which essentially eliminated all medical research in the field for almost 30 years. This action was tragic for science, as chemists were extremely close to isolating the active chemical ingredient of marijuana prior to World War II. The identification of delta-9-tetrahydrocannabinol (THC) had to wait for the elegant efforts of Raphael Mechoulam in the 1960s.

This pattern of a few steps forward followed by a few steps backward in how societies deal with marijuana has been repeated even in the seven-year interval between the first and second editions of this volume. When I wrote the foreword to the first edition, the science of marijuana was burgeoning. Identification of putative endogenous ligands for the cannabinoid receptors portended the development of simple drug-like chemicals that might mimic or block these receptors with therapeutic application. In the past seven years, the science has accelerated so that one might have anticipated more enlightened legal approaches to the medical uses of marijuana.

Several American states did provide enabling legislation. By contrast, the U.S. Justice Department ruled that all such uses were illegal. Thus physicians in California and other states prescribing the drug in accordance with state law would be vulnerable to federal prosecution.

What are some of the principal scientific advances over the past seven years? In the 1990s, Mechoulam had isolated endogenous brain constituents that mimicked THC in terms of its pharmacologic actions and interactions with cannabinoid receptors. These were postulated to be "endocannabinoids," the brain's own marijuana-like neurotransmitters or neuromodulators in analogy to the endorphins and opiate receptors. However, it is extremely difficult to prove definitively that a given brain chemical is the substance that normally regulates a particular receptor. Compelling evidence has now accumulated to establish that the materials isolated by Mechoulam are normally involved in regulating cannabinoid receptors. Enzymes that degrade and presumably inactivate the endocannabinoids have been isolated, and drugs that inhibit these enzymes elicit marijuana-like actions in animals.

Thus, we now are reasonably confident that there exist endocannabinoids that are important regulators of brain function. Work in the past few years has pinned down how such agents act. Studies by Roger Nicoll and others have shown that the direction in which endocannabinoids signal between neurons is "backward" to conventional neurotransmitters. They provide retrograde signaling from "receiving" neurons to the "sending" neurons. These discoveries have been made possible by using novel cannabinoid receptor antagonist drugs, of which one, rimonabant, is already on the market in several European countries. The development of rimonabant and the likely emergence of other cannabinoid receptor drugs represent the second major advance of the past decade. One would expect such a drug to elicit effects opposite to those caused by marijuana. All marijuana users get "the munchies," developing robust appetites. Indeed, for centuries in India marijuana extracts were widely prescribed to stimulate appetite. The initial therapeutic objective of rimonabant is to do the opposite, to decrease appetite and body weight. One would also expect rimonabant to elicit symptoms opposite to other actions of marijuana, which causes a calm, good feeling. The principal side effects of rimonabant are anxiety and depression.

Though their incidence is relatively low, such effects would be worrisome for a drug likely to be used by vast numbers of individuals desiring to lose a few pounds. As of this writing the advisory committee to the United States Food and Drug Administration has recommended that rimonibant not be approved for marketing.

The first edition of this volume was of immense value to the intelligent reader, as it presented the facts about marijuana lucidly and in a remarkably easy-to-read literary style. For the second edition, Dr. Iversen has again provided a book that is a pleasurable must-read for anyone who cares about drugs and society. He has updated all the science, social, and legal facets of marijuana study. I am confident that you, like I, will adore this fine volume.

# *Preface to the Second Edition*

As a scientist who works on understanding how drugs act on the brain, I continue to be exasperated by the way in which science is used and abused by the proponents and opponents of cannabis in defending their positions. This is a drug whose actions have been studied in some detail; there is a considerable scientific literature on how it acts and the possible adverse effects associated with its long-term use. Millions of young people on both sides of the Atlantic are more or less regular users of cannabis, but official attitudes vary widely. In Europe several countries have relaxed the legal penalties associated with its use. But in the United States cannabis continues to be viewed as the number one drug problem, and accounts for more than three quarters of a million arrests each year—often followed by draconian penalties.

There have been exciting new scientific advances in the past few years with the discovery that the brain contains its own "cannabis-like" chemical messenger system—a finding potentially as important as the much publicized discovery of a naturally occurring series of morphine-like chemicals in the brain—the endorphins—in the 1970s. Research in this new field has grown rapidly since the first edition of this book was published. Less than 200 scientific papers had been published by then on these newly discovered chemicals, but more than 2,000 additional publications have appeared since. There is an increasing understanding that the naturally occurring cannabis system plays many roles in the body apart from acting as modulators of neural activity in the brain (see Chapter 3).

## Pub Med Citations

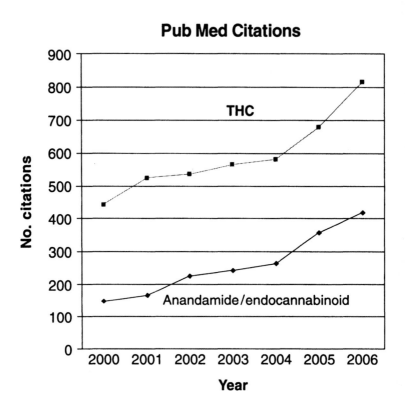

In July 1996 the British Minister of Health, in reply to a Parliamentary question about the medical uses of cannabis, said, "At present the evidence is inconclusive. The key point is that a cannabis-based medicine has not been scientifically demonstrated to be safe, efficacious and of suitable quality." In August of that year General Barry McCaffrey, the U.S. drug czar, somewhat more bluntly said, "There is not a shred of scientific evidence that shows that smoked marijuana is useful or needed. This is not medicine. This is a cruel hoax." But time has shown them both to be wrong. There have been important advances in the medical applications of cannabis in the last few years, with the first large-scale clinical trials of cannabis-based medicines and the approval of one such prescription medicine in Canada.

Meanwhile, the new scientific knowledge of naturally occurring cannabi-noids in the body has offered entirely new approaches to the discovery and development of novel cannabinoid-based medicines.

Altogether, the past 6 years have seen an exciting transformation of cannabis research from the study of a plant-derived psychoactive drug (delta-9-tetrahydrocannabinol) (THC) to a flourishing new field of basic medical research that offers great scientific and medical promise for the future.

L.I.
Oxford, U.K.
2007

# Contents

Foreword, v

1  Introduction, 3

The Plant, 6
Consumption of Cannabis: Preparations for Their
Psychoactive Effects, 13
    *Smoking, 14*
    *Eating and Drinking, 15*
A Brief History, 17

2  The Pharmacology of Delta-9-Tetrahydrocannabinol
(THC), The Psychoactive Ingredient in Cannabis, 27

Man-Made Cannabinoids, 36
Cannabinoid Antagonists, 39
How Does THC Get to the Brain? 41
    *Smoking, 41*
    *Oral Absorption, 43*
    *Other Routes of Administration, 46*
Elimination of THC From the Body, 47
How Does THC Work? 48
    *Discovery of Cannabinoid Receptors, 48*
    *Neuroanatomical Distribution of CB-1 Receptors in the Brain, 54*

Some Physiological Effects of THC, 56
*Inhibition of Neurotransmitter Release, 56*
*Effects on the Heart and Blood Vessels, 57*
*Effects on Pain Sensitivity, 59*
*Effects on Motility and Posture, 61*
*The Billy Martin Tetrad, 64*

3 Endocannabinoids, 67

Discovery of Naturally Occurring Endocannabinoids—
The Endocannabinoids, 68
Biosynthesis and Inactivation of Endocannabinoids, 70
Physiological Functions of Endocannabinoids, 72
*Retrograde Signal Molecules at Synapses, 72*
*Control of Energy Metabolism and Body Weight, 74*
*Regulation of Pain Sensitivity, 74*
*Cardiovascular Control, 76*
*Other Functions, 76*
Development of a New Endocannabinoid-Based Pharmacology, 77
*Novel Cannabinoid Receptor Agonists or Antagonists, 77*
*Inhibitors of Endocannabinoid Inactivation, 77*

4 The Effects of Cannabis on the Central Nervous System, 81

Subjective Reports of the Marijuana High, 82
Laboratory Studies of Marijuana in Human Volunteers, 94
*Effects on Movement and Driving, 95*
*Higher Brain Function, Including Learning and Memory, 96*
*Comparisons of Marijuana With Alcohol, 98*
What Can Animal Behavior Experiments Tell Us? 99
Does Repeated Use of Marijuana Lead to
Tolerance and Dependence? 105

5 Medical Uses of Marijuana—Fact or Fantasy? 115

Historical, 116

The Modern Revival of Interest in Cannabis-Based Medicines, 122
The Synthetic Cannabinoids, 128
  *Dronabinol (Marinol),* 129
  *Nabilone (Cesamet),* 130
Medical Targets for Cannabis, 131
  *Multiple Sclerosis,* 131
  *Pain,* 137
  *Nausea and Vomiting Associated With Cancer Chemotherapy,* 141
  *AIDS Wasting Syndrome,* 144
  *Other Potential Medical Targets,* 145
    Epilepsy, 145
    Bronchial Asthma, 146
    Moods Disorders and Sleep, 147
    Cancer, 148
    Diarrhea, 148
    Emerging Indications, 148
Is There Any Role for Smoked Marijuana as a Medicine? 149
A Cannabinoid Antagonist for the Treatment of Obesity, 151
  *Preclinical Data,* 151
  *Clinical Data,* 152
Conclusions, 155


6  Is Cannabis Safe? 157

Toxicity, 158
Acute Effects of Cannabis, 162
Effects of Long-Term Exposure to Cannabis, 164
  *Are There Persistent Cognitive Deficits?* 164
  *Tolerance and Dependence,* 167
  *Adverse Effects on Fertility and the Unborn Child,* 168
  *Suppression of Immune System Function,* 170
  *Cannabis and Mental Illness,* 171
Special Hazards of Smoked Marijuana, 175
  *Marijuana Smoke and Smoking Behavior,* 175
  *Effects of Marijuana Smoke on the Lungs,* 179
  *Marijuana Smoking and Lung Cancer,* 181
Summary, 185

7   The Recreational Use of Cannabis, 187

Prevalence, 189
How Is Cannabis Consumed and Where Does It Come From? 192
Patterns of Recreational Use, 195
What Are the Effects of Recreational Cannabis Use? 198
The Potency of Illicit Marijuana, 201
Is Marijuana a Gateway Drug? 206
Do Recreational Marijuana Users Become Dependent? 209
Forensic Testing for Cannabis—Growth Industry, 212
Snapshots of Cannabis Use Around the World, 214
    *India and Pakistan,* 214
    *Nepal and Tibet,* 216
    *Southeast Asia,* 216
    *Africa,* 217
    *Caribbean and Latin America,* 217
Conclusions, 219


8   What Next? A Hundred Years of Cannabis Reports, 221

A Hundred Years of Cannabis Inquiries, 223
    *The Indian Hemp Drugs Commission Report (1894),* 223
    *Mayor La Guardia's Report,* The Marihuana Problem
    in the City of New York *(1944),* 225
    The Wooton Report, *England (1969),* 227
    *Report Followed Report,* 229
The Dutch Experiment, 232
What Next? Is There a Case for the Legalization/Decriminalization/
Depenalization of Cannabis? 238


References, 243
Index, 261

*The Science*
*of*
*Marijuana*

# 1

## *Introduction*

Marijuana (cannabis) is among the most widely used of all psychoactive drugs. Despite the fact that its possession and use is illegal in most countries, cannabis is used regularly by as many as 20 million people in the United States and Europe and by millions more in other parts of the world. Thousands of patients with AIDS, multiple sclerosis, and a variety of other disabling diseases illegally smoke marijuana with the firm belief that it makes their symptoms better, despite the relative paucity of medical evidence to substantiate this. A great deal of new evidence for the medical benefits of cannabis has been obtained recently from carefully controlled clinical trials, however, and it is likely that cannabis-based medicines will gain official approval in many countries soon, as has already happened in Canada.

Since 1996 voters in 12 states in the United States (Alaska, California, Colorado, Hawaii, Maine, Maryland, Montana, Nevada, Oregon, Rhode Island, Vermont, and Washington) have approved propositions making marijuana available for medical use with a doctor's recommendation. Cannabis buyers clubs or pharmacies have been established in these states to provide supplies of cannabis for medicinal use. On the whole, these are run by well-intentioned people and are strictly regulated. Patients are checked for identity, medical records, and doctor's diagnosis before they are allowed to purchase small quantities of marijuana.

The Netherlands pioneered the separation of cannabis from "hard" drugs such as cocaine or heroin in the 1970s, and established licensed "coffee shops" for the legal supply of small quantities of cannabis. In Amsterdam, the Blue Velvet Coffee Shop is a typical example, located on a busy city street, adjacent to shops and cafes. Inside it seems to be a small, friendly, and ordinary place, one of more than 700 similar establishments in Dutch cities. There are a few posters on the wall, a coin-operated video game, and loud music. Behind the bar, along with the usual espresso machine and soft drinks, is the menu, which features 30 varieties of cannabis resin and 28 varieties of marijuana leaf. Customers come in to purchase a small *bag* or some *hash brownies* to take away, and some linger to smoke marijuana joints on the premises while drinking their cappuccino. Regular customers have their loyalty card stamped with each purchase (one bag free as a bonus for every four purchased).

There are some indications that Western society is starting to take a more liberal view toward cannabis use, one that tends toward the Dutch assessment of it as a "soft" drug that should be distinguished and separated from hard drugs. But fierce opposition to cannabis use remains in many quarters. The U.S. federal government continues to view cannabis as a dangerous drug and imposes harsh penalties for possession or dealing. The federal government has tried repeatedly (and so far unsuccessfully) to close the cannabis buyers clubs in California and in other states and has threatened to punish both doctors and their patients for their involvement in this illegal drug use. In Europe, reports that teenage cannabis use might lead to mental illness in later life have gained a great deal of prominence (see Chapter 7), and in Britain this led to a move in 2006 to reconsider the legal downgrading of cannabis, which had taken place in 2004, although in the end the downgrading remained.

Even in liberal Holland, the coffee shops have no legal means of obtaining their supplies of cannabis, and the Dutch government is under considerable pressure from nearby European countries to modify its policy. With the absence of customs borders in the European Union, it is very easy for people from neighboring France, Germany, or Belgium to stock up on cannabis from Dutch outlets. There are strong political moves to limit access to the coffee shops to Dutch nationals only.

Who is right? Is cannabis a relatively harmless "soft" drug? Does it have genuine medical uses that cannot be fulfilled by other medicines? Or is the campaign to legalize the medical use of cannabis merely a smoke-screen used by those seeking the wider acceptance of the drug? Is cannabis in fact an addictive narcotic drug that governments are right to protect the public from? This book will review the scientific and medical evidence on cannabis and try to answer some of these questions. Often, in analyzing the mass of scientific data, it is difficult to come to clear-cut conclusions. To make matters worse in this particular case, the opposing factions in the cannabis debate often interpret the same scientific evidence differently to suit their own purposes.

This introductory chapter will introduce the hemp plant from which the various cannabis products derive and will give a brief history of the drug.

## The Plant

The hemp plant (*Cannabis sativa*) probably originated in Central Asia but has been distributed widely around the world through man's activities (for a comprehensive review of cannabis botany see Clarke, 1981). It has been cultivated as a multipurpose economic plant for thousands of years, and through the process of selection for various desirable characteristics many different cultivated varieties exist—some grown exclusively for their fiber content, others for their content of psychoactive chemicals. All of these varieties, however, are generally classified as a single species first named in 1735 by the famous Swedish botanist Linnaeus as *Cannabis sativa*. The Cannabis plant is a lush, fast-growing annual, which can reach maturity in 60 days when grown indoors under optimum heat and light conditions and in 3 to 5 months in outdoor cultivation. The plant has characteristic finely branched leaves subdivided into lance-shaped leaflets with a saw-tooth edge. The woody, angular, hairy stem may reach a height of 15 feet or more under optimum conditions. A smaller, more bushy subspecies reaching only 4 feet or so in height known as *Cannabis indica* was first described by Lamark and is recognized by some modern botanists. There has been much activity among plant breeders in Holland (where cultivation of the plant for personal use is legal) and in California (where such cultivation is illegal) to produce new varieties with increased yields of the psychoactive chemical delta-9-tetrahydrocannabinol (THC). The details of the breeding programs are not public, but involve such techniques as the treatment of cannabis seed with the chemical colchicine to cause the creation of polyploid plants, in which each cell contains multiple sets of chromosomes instead of the normal single set. Such varieties may have extra vigor and an enhanced production of THC, although they tend to be genetically unstable. Other varieties have been obtained by crossing *Cannabis sativa* with *Cannabis indica* strains, to yield a number of different hybrids. These strains may not breed true, but by selecting the first-generation (F1 hybrid) seeds of such crosses plants can be generated with hybrid vigor and enhanced THC production. Particularly favorable genetic strains can also be propagated vegetatively by cuttings—in this way a single plant can give rise to thousands of clones with identical genetic makeup to the original.

Although the cultivation of cannabis for THC production is illegal in most Western countries, the Internet carries advertisements from numerous seed companies, which offer to supply seeds of as many as 30 different varieties of cannabis—with such names as Skunk, Northern Lights, Amstel Gold, and Early Girl. Prices for individual seeds average US $5, but in something approaching the seventeenth-century "tulipmania" Dutch suppliers seek as much as US $15 to $20 for a single seed of varieties such as Arjan's Ultra Haze #1 Greenhouse, which won the High Times Cup in the 2006 Amsterdam Cannabis Festival and which, according to the seed supplier, is said to generate a "very intense sativa high, a real blast, a very psychedelic feeling."

The cannabis plant is either male or female, and under normal growing conditions these are generated in roughly equal numbers. The male plant produces an obvious flower head, which produces pollen, while the female flower heads are less obvious and contain the ovaries ensheathed in green bracts and hairs (Fig. 1.1). The psychoactive chemical THC is present in most parts of the plant, including the leaves and flowers, but it is most highly concentrated in fine droplets of sticky resin produced by glands at the base of the fine hairs, which coat the leaves and particularly the bracts of the female flower head. The resin may act as a natural varnish, coating the leaves and flowers to protect them from desiccation in the hot, dry conditions in which the plant often grows. Contrary to the ancient belief that only the female plant produces THC, the leaves of male and female plants contain approximately the same amounts of THC, although the male plant lacks the highly concentrated THC content associated with the female flowers. If pollinated, the female flower head will develop seeds; these contain no THC but have a high nutritional value. Indeed, cannabis was an important food crop—listed as one of the five major grains in ancient China—and is still cultivated for this purpose in some parts of the world today. From the point of view of the cannabis smoker, however, the presence of seeds is undesirable: they burn with an acrid smoke and tend to explode on heating, and their presence dilutes the THC content of the female flower head. In the cultivation of cannabis for drug use in India, it was customary to remove all the male plants from the crop as they began to flower to yield the resin-rich sterile female

A

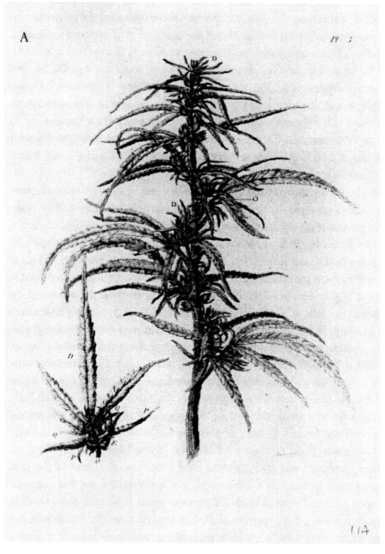

**Figure 1.1.** Engravings showing the characteristic appearance of the flowering heads of female (*A*) and male (*B*) cannabis plants. (From Wisset, 1808.)

B

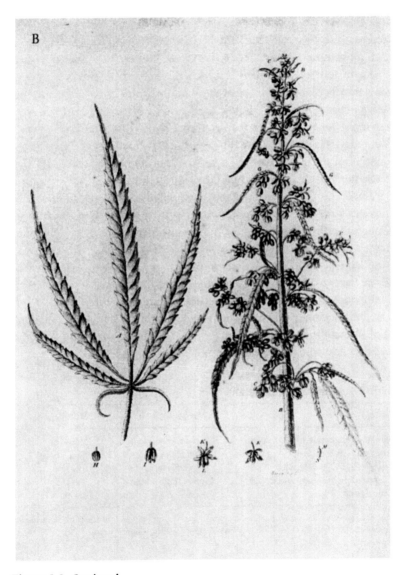

**Figure 1.1.** *Continued*

flowering heads, which were dried and compressed to form the potent product known as *ganja*. The services of expert *ganja doctors* were often employed, who went through the hemp field with an expert eye cutting down all the male plants before they could flower. The labor-intensive process of removing all male plants is rarely used by Western growers today; female plants can be cultivated simply by taking cuttings or using seed genetically modified to produce female-only plants. The dried sterile female flower heads are known as *sensimilla* (sometimes *sensemilla*). These may contain up to five times more THC than the *marijuana*[1] produced from the dried leaves of other parts of the plant (Table 1.1). The most potent preparation derived directly from the plant is *hashish*, which represents the THC-rich cannabis resin obtained by scraping the resin from the flower heads or by rubbing the dried flower heads and leaves through a series of sieves to obtain the dried particles of resin sometimes misleadingly known as *pollen* (which, strictly speaking, can only come from male plants). These are compressed to form a cake of yellow to dark brown hashish known as *resin* or the higher quality finely sieved *polm*. The process not only reduces the space required for storage, but also ensures longer storage life by reducing potential deterioration of herbal material through rot, mold, or infestation. The solid block of resin becomes sealed in its own oxidized coating.

**Table 1.1.** Cannabis Preparations

| Name | Part of Plant | THC Content (%) |
|---|---|---|
| Marijuana (cannabis, bhang, dagga, kif) | Leaves, small stems | 4.0–6.0 |
| Sensimilla (sensemilla) | Female flower heads | 9.0–12.0 |
| Resin (hashish, charas, polm) | Cannabis resin* | 10.0–15.0* |
| Cultivated plants (skunk, *nederwiet*) | Indoor cultivation | 10.0–20.0 |
| Cannabis oil | Alcoholic resin extract | 20.0–60.0 |

* Street samples of cannabis resin often contain much smaller quantities of THC because they are frequently adulterated with other substances; an average of 5% THC would be typical.

1. The term *marijuana* is widely used in North America to describe herbal cannabis; in Europe the word *cannabis* is more common. In this book the two words will be used interchangeably.

A more colorful method of obtaining the pure resin in India was described in 1840 by the Irish doctor William B. O'Shaugnessy, who worked for many years in India:

> Men clad in leather dresses run through the hemp field, brushing through the plants with all possible violence; the soft resin adheres to the leather, is subsequently scraped off and kneaded into balls, which sell from five to six rupees the seer. A still finer kind...is collected by hand in Nepal—the leather attire is dispensed with, and the resin is gathered on the skins of naked coolies. (O'Shaugnessey, 1842)

Another product is *cannabis oil*, produced by repeatedly extracting hashish resin with alcohol. The concentrated alcoholic extract may vary in color from green (if prepared from resin containing significant amounts of fresh cannabis leaf) to yellow or colorless for the purer preparations. It can contain up to an alarmingly high 60% THC content, but more usually the THC content is around 20%. Nevertheless, one drop of such oil can contain as much THC as a single marijuana cigarette.

The cannabis plant develops in many different ways, according to the genetic variety and the soil, temperature, and lighting conditions under which it is grown. To generate optimum quantities of THC, the plant needs a fertile soil and long hours of daylight, preferably in a sunny and warm climate. This means essentially that for THC production, growth occurs optimally anywhere within 35 degrees of the equator. Typical growing regions include Mexico, northern India, and many parts of Africa, Afghanistan, and California. In northern Europe and Russia the plant has long been cultivated as a fiber crop, but such plants are grown from varieties selected for this purpose and do not generate significant amounts of THC.

Nowadays, the culture of cannabis often takes place indoors, where nutrients, lighting, and temperature conditions can be optimized and the cultivation (illegal in most countries) can be more easily concealed. More than half of the cannabis consumed in the coffee shops in the Netherlands is grown domestically under indoor conditions. Illegal cannabis *farms* have multiplied on both sides of the Atlantic—often using a private house in which all the windows have been covered to conceal the intense lighting and where the meter has been bypassed to tap directly into the main electricity supply to conceal the large amounts of power used. Plants are grown on specially enriched soils or with hydroponics, and their growth cycle has been shortened to less than 4 months. The product has a higher THC content than traditional imported cannabis. It is estimated that as much as 50% of European cannabis consumption is accounted for by indigenous production, and this is expanding rapidly. The increased availability of such artificially cultivated cannabis has led to concerns that this higher potency material may be more dangerous than old-fashioned marijuana. But the highest potency cultivated cannabis available (10% to 20% THC) compares with the THC content of herbal marijauna or resin at around 5%. The cultivated forms of cannabis are thus 2–4 times more potent, not 10- to 20-fold as often claimed. But the warnings about superpotent cannabis have become firmly embedded as a media myth, accepted by reputable newspapers and even by the British Broadcasting Corporation as an established truth. In Britain the situation was exacerbated by a report on cannabis issued by the Royal College of General Practitioners, which warned that a cannabis joint today could contain as much as 300 mg THC by comparison with about 10 mg previously. This is clearly impossible, as the average joint only contains a total of around 500 mg of herbal cannabis or resin—but the report was seen by all 50,000 physicians in Britain! The Royal College subsequently corrected its mistake—but by then it was too late.

The large variability in THC production according to strain and culture conditions presents one of the problems associated with the use of herbal cannabis as a medicinal or recreational drug; the consumer of an illegal and uncontrolled plant material has little indication of its THC content, and may consequently fail to obtain an adequate dose or, alternatively, may unwittingly take a larger dose than desired.

The cannabis plant is nowadays thought of mainly in the context of the psychoactive drug THC, but it is a versatile species that has had a very important place in human agriculture for thousands of years (for reviews see Robinson, 1996; Russo, 2007). An acre of hemp produces more cellulose than an acre of trees, and the tough fiber produced from the outer layers of the stem has had many important uses. Hemp fiber made the ropes that lifted up the tough hemp-derived canvas cloth (the word derives from the Dutch pronunciation of cannabis) used to make the sails of the ancient Phoenician, Greek, and Roman navies. Archeological evidence shows that hemp fiber production was going on in northeastern Asia in Neolithic times, around 600 B.C., and hemp production spread around the world, including the United States, where it was introduced by the first settlers. Although the importance of hemp declined with years, there were still 42,000 acres cultivated in the United States in 1917. Other major commercial centers of production were in Europe and in Russia. Ships' sails, ropes, clothing, towels, and paper were all derived from hemp fiber and the woody cellulose-rich interior *hurds* of the hemp stem. Until the 1880s, almost all of the world's paper was made from hemp, and even today many bank notes are still printed on cannabis paper because of its toughness and durability. Most of our great artwork is painted on canvas, and the first Levi jeans were made from canvas cloth.

Robert Wisset in his *Treatise on Hemp* (1808) gave a comprehensive account of the cultivation of hemp as a fiber plant in Europe, Asia, and America two centuries ago.

Hemp seed has also been an important food crop, and from it can be derived oil, which has many uses as a lubricant, paint ingredient, ink solvent, and cooking oil. The seeds are now used mainly for animal feed and as birdseed.

Most of the ancient uses of hemp have been overtaken by the advent of cotton goods, synthetic fibers, forestry-derived paper, and alternative food grains. Nevertheless, the cultivation of hemp as a fiber crop still continues on a small scale in Europe. With the sanction of the European Union, farms in Hampshire in Southern England, a traditional center for hemp farming, continue to grow the crop.

## Consumption of Cannabis: Preparations for Their Psychoactive Effects

Cannabis products have been consumed for thousands of years in different human cultures. It is not surprising that this has taken many different forms, and only some of the more common will be described here.

## Smoking

Smoking is one of the most efficient ways of ingesting cannabis and rapidly experiencing its effects on the brain (Chapter 2). The favorite of many people in the West is the marijuana joint. This consists of a variable quantity of dried marijuana leaf (from which stems and seeds have first carefully been removed) rolled inside a rice-paper cylinder either by hand or using a rolling machine. A typical joint would contain about a half gram of leaf with or without added tobacco—which assists the otherwise often erratic burning of the marijuana. Many different slang words describe herbal marijuana, for example: Aunt Mary, dope, grass, joint, Mary Jane, reefer, spliff, and weed. When a joint has been smoked down to the point that it is difficult to hold it is called a *roach,* and this still contains appreciable amounts of THC, which gradually distills down the length of the joint as it is smoked. The roach may be held in the split end of a match or with a variety of *roach pins* or tweezers with which one may hold the roach without burning oneself. In the social groups in which marijuana is commonly smoked, as with the port served in Oxford and Cambridge Colleges after dinner, etiquette demands that the joint is passed around the group in a circular fashion. As with the port, hoarding of the joint by any one person is regarded as a serious breach of protocol. Experienced marijuana smokers often develop the technique of inhaling a considerable quantity of air along with the smoke—this dilutes the smoke, making it less irritating to the airways and allowing deeper inhalation. Marijuana smokers tend to inhale more deeply than cigarette smokers do and hold the air in their lungs for longer before exhaling.

Marijuana can also be smoked using a variety of pipes. A simple pipe resembling those used for tobacco can be used, but marijuana pipes are usually made of such heat-resistant materials as stone, glass, ivory, or metal. This is necessary because marijuana does not tend to stay alight in a pipe so it constantly has to be relit. A common variety of pipe is the water pipe or bong. These come in many different forms but all use the same principle. Smoke from the pipe is sucked through a layer of water, which cools it and removes much of the tar and other irritant materials present in marijuana leaf smoke. Bongs tend to be complex and heavy devices and thus not easily portable.

The more potent forms of cannabis, sensemilla, ganja, and cannabis resin are also often smoked using cigarettes or a pipe, and commonly
mixed with tobacco. Pipe smoking is the traditional method for smoking
ganja in India and hashish in the Arab world. Khwaja A. Hasan gives the
following description of ganja smoking in contemporary India:

> Ganja is smoked in a funnel-shaped clay pipe called chilam. Almost anybody
> except the untouchables (sweeper caste) can join the group and enjoy a few
> puffs. The base part of the bowl portion of the funnel-shaped pipe is first cov-
> ered with a small charred clay filter. Then the mixture of ganja and tobacco
> is placed on this filter. A small ring, the size of the bowl, of rope fibre called
> baand is first burnt separately and then quickly placed on top of the smoking
> material. The pipe is now ready for smoking. Usually four or five people gather
> around a pipe.... Ritual purity of the pipe is always preserved for the clay pipe
> is never touched by the lips of the smoker. The tubular part of the chilam at its
> bottom is held in the right hand and the left hand also supports it. The passage
> between the index finger and the thumb of the right hand is used in taking
> puffs from the pipe.... While they sit in a squatting position on a chabootra
> (raised platform) in front of one person's house, or gather in an open space
> while the host prepares the chilam they talk about social problems, weather,
> crops, prices, marriage negotiations and so forth. Such gatherings may take
> place at any time during the day except early morning. After a smoke they
> again go back to work. Thus such smoking parties are like "coffee breaks" in
> the American culture. (Hasan, see Rubin, 1975)

In modern Western society the use of cannabis oil has been introduced (a very potent alcoholic extract of cannabis resin). A few drops of this
added to a normal tobacco cigarette offers a means of smoking cannabis
that is hard to detect.

## Eating and Drinking

THC is soluble in fats and in alcohol so it can be extracted and added to
various foodstuffs and drinks and taken into the body in that way. This
method of consumption gives a much slower absorption (see Chapter 2)
and avoids the irritant effects of inhaled smoke that many people find

objectionable. The heating of marijuana during the preparation of food-stuffs or drinks leads to the formation of additional THC from the chemical breakdown of pharmacologically inactive carboxylic acid THC derivatives present in the plant preparations. A common method is to heat the plant leaf in butter, margarine, or cooking oil and then to strain out the solid plant materials and use the oil or butter for cooking—often to make cakes and biscuits (e.g., hash brownies). THC can also be extracted with alcohol by heating and straining, yielding a variety of tinctures (e.g., Green Dragon), which can be diluted with lemonade or other flavored drinks. In the former United States and British medical use of cannabis, the formulations used were alcoholic extracts of the plant, sometimes diluted further with alcohol to yield *tincture of cannabis*. This was diluted with water and administered by mouth.

In India, smoking marijuana in the form of cigarettes has never been popular. *Bhang* (marijuana) is commonly rolled into small balls and eaten, or infused in boiling water with or without added milk to form a drink. Such methods yield preparations with only modest amounts of THC—as the active compound is not water soluble. The fats present in milk, however, make this a more effective means of extracting THC. In Indian cities bhang is sometimes added to the milk used for making an ice cream called *gulfi*. Many different cannabis-containing drinks and foods are known in Indian culture. Khwaja A. Hasan gives the following description of the famous decoction prepared from bhang called *thandai:*

> Preparing thandai is a time-consuming process. A number of dry fruits, condiments and spices are used in its preparation. Almonds, pistachio, rose petals, black pepper, aniseed, and cloves are ground on the toothed grinding plate (silauti); water is added so that a thinly ground paste is obtained. This paste is dissolved in milk and then bhang is added to the mixture. A few spoons of sugar or jaggery (boiled brown sugar) are added finally and then the decoction is ready for consumption.... The preparation of thandai and the social atmosphere it creates has great significance. Members of the same family, caste or a circle of friends from the village or the neighbourhood gather in the parlour of a friend. Different ingredients of the drink are collected and ground on the toothed stone grinding plate. The whole process takes an hour or so. While preparing the drink, individuals talk about friends,

family members, prices of goods and services and a host of other problems. (Hasan, see Rubin, 1975)

Around the world a variety of different cannabis preparations have been devised in different cultures and the diversity of this range equals the many different forms in which human beings have traditionally consumed alcohol—from light beer to distilled spirits, from vin de table to Premier Cru chateau-bottled clarets.

## A Brief History

Excellent reviews of the long history of cannabis can be found in Abel (1943), Lewin (1931), Robinson (1996), Walton (1938), Booth (2003), and Russo (2007). Evidence of man's first use of cannabis has been found in fragments of pottery bearing the imprint of a cord-like material thought to be of hemp in Taiwan, dated around 10,000 B.C. Other early evidence for hemp cultivation comes from the finding of fragments of hemp cloth in Chinese burial chambers from the Chou dynasty (1122–265 B.C). It seems likely that hemp was cultivated and used for the manufacture of ropes, nets, canvas sails, and cloths in ancient China. The first descriptions of the medical and intoxicant properties of the plant are to be found in the ancient Chinese herbal *Pen-ts'ao*, ca. 1–2 century AD. Classical myth relates that the Chinese deity Shen Nung tested hundreds of herbal materials in a series of heroic experiments in self-medication and agronomics. So potent was this myth of the etiology of medicine that the god's name was attached to the Pen-ts'ao. This herbal pharmacopoeia describes hundreds of drugs, among them cannabis, which was called *ma*, a pun for "chaotic." This ancient text clearly describes the stupefying and hallucinogenic properties of the plant. Pharmacologists and herbalists added sections to the text for many centuries and Chinese physicians used cumulative editions of Pen-ts'ao as the standard text on medical drugs for hundreds of years. Shen Nung, the farmer god, became the patron deity of medicine, with the title "Father of Chinese Medicine." Ma, often mixed with wine in a preparation called *ma-yao*, was used principally for its pain-relieving properties. Although there seems also to have been some use of the drug as an intoxicant in China, this never became widespread.

In contrast to China, the use of cannabis for its psychoactive properties has been endemic in India for more than a thousand years. Cannabis use was known by the nomadic tribes of northeastern Asia in Neolithic times, and may have played an important role in the practice of the religion of shamanism by these people. The nomads brought the plant and its uses to Western Asia and then to India. Ancient Indian legend tells how the Hindu god Siva became angry after a family row and wandered off into the fields by himself. Exhausted by the heat of the sun, he sought shade and refuge under a leafy plant and finally went to sleep. On waking he became curious about the plant that had given him shelter and ate some of its leaves. This made him feel so refreshed that he adopted it as his favorite food. From then on Siva was known as the Lord of bhang. In ancient Indian texts bhang is referred to in the *Science of Charms*—written between 2000 and 1400 B.C.—as one of the "five kingdoms of herbs...which release us from anxiety." Bhang seems to have been popular with the Indian people from the beginning of history. The Indian Hemp Drugs Commission Report (1894) gave a detailed picture of how bhang and the more potent cannabis products ganja and charas (the Indian term for cannabis resin) had become incorporated into Indian life and culture.

It took longer for cannabis to reach the West. Hemp was known to the Assyrian civilization both as a fiber plant and a medicine and is referred to as *kunnubu* or *kunnapu* in Assyrian documents of around 600 B.C. The word is probably the basis of the Arabian *kinnab* and the Greek and Latin *cannabis*. There is little evidence that the plant was known beyond Turkey until the time of the Greeks. The Greeks used hemp for the manufacture of ropes and sails for their conquering navies, as did the Romans later— although the hemp was not cultivated in Greece or Italy but in the further reaches of their empires in Asia Minor. Neither the Greeks nor the Romans, however, appear to have used cannabis for its psychoactive properties, although these were known and described by the Roman physicians Dioscorides, Galen, and Oribasius. Galen, writing in the second century A.D., described how wealthy Romans sometimes offered their dinner guests an exotic dessert containing cannabis seeds:

> There are those who eat it (cannabis seed) also cooked with other confec-
> tions, by this confection is meant a sort of dessert which is taken after meals
> with drinks for the purpose of exciting pleasure. It creates much warmth (or
> possibly excitement) and when taken too generously affects the head emit-
> ting a warm vapor and acting as a drug. (Walton, 1938, p. 8)

As the seeds contain no significant amounts of psychoactive material, it
seems likely that some other parts of the cannabis plant must also have
been included.

It was to be almost another thousand years before cannabis spread to
the Arab lands and then to Europe and the Americas. According to one
Arab legend, the discovery of marijuana dates back to the twelfth century
AD when a monk and recluse named Hayder, a Persian founder of the religious order of Sufi, came across the plant while wandering in meditation
in the mountains. When he returned to his monastery after eating some
cannabis leaves, his disciples were amazed at how talkative and animated
this normally dour and taciturn man had become. After they persuaded
Hayder to tell them what had made him so happy, the disciples went out
into the mountains and tried some cannabis themselves. By the thirteenth
century, cannabis use had become common in the Arab lands, giving rise
to many colorful legends. Bhang and hashish are referred to frequently in
the *Arabian Nights* or *The Thousand and One Nights* folk tales collected
during the period 1000 to 1700 A.D.:

> Furthermore, I conceive that the twain are eaters of Hashish, which
> drug when swallowed by man, maketh him prattle of whatso he pleaseth
> and chooseth, making him now a Sultan, then a Wazir, and then a mer-
> chant, the while it seemeth to him that the world is in the hollow of his
> hand. Tis composed of hemp leaflets whereto are added aromatic roots
> and somewhat of sugar; then they cook it and prepare a kind of confec-
> tion which they eat, but whoso eateh it (especially if he eat more than
> enough) talketh of matters which reason may on no wise represent. (Wal-
> ton, 1938, p. 15)

It is clear from this description that the word *hashish* in ancient Arab writings refers to what we would now call marijuana rather than the cannabis

resin that the term hashish now describes. Outstanding among the Arab legends is the story of the *Old Man of the Mountains* and his murderous band of followers known as the *Assassins*. According to Marco Polo, who recorded this legend, the Assassins were led by the Old Man of the Mountains who recruited novices to his band and kept them under his control as his docile servants by feeding them copious amounts of hashish. Marco Polo described how the leader constructed a remarkable garden at his major fortress, the Alamut. The young assassins would be transported to the garden after they had taken enough hashish to put them to sleep. When they awoke, and found themselves in such a beautiful place with ladies willing to dally with them to their heart's content, they believed that they were indeed in paradise. When the Old Man wanted someone killed, he would tell the assassins to do it and promise them that, dead or alive, they would return to paradise; they obeyed his commands with great brutality.

Although the historical facts are impossible to determine, it seems likely that the Assassins were led by Hasan-Ibn-Sabbah, who started life as a religious missionary and later gathered a secret band of followers. They probably used hashish, as did many others in the Arab world at that time. It does not seem likely that they would have been able to carry out their terrorist acts or politically motivated assassinations while intoxicated by cannabis, nor is there any significant evidence that the drug inspires violence — on the contrary, it tends to cause somnolence and lethargy when taken in high doses. Nevertheless, lurid stories about the drug-crazed Assassins have been widely used in the West as part of the mythology that surrounds the cannabis debate. As early as the twelfth century, Abbot Arnold of Lübeck wrote in *Chronica Slavorum*:

> Hemp raises them to a state of ecstasy or folly, or intoxicates them. Then sorcerers draw near and exhibit to the sleepers phantasms, pleasures and amusements. They then promise that these delights will become perpetual if the orders given them are executed with the daggers provided.

Eight hundred years later in the United States, the hard-line commissioner of the Federal Bureau of Narcotics, Harry J. Anslinger, used the image of the drug-crazed Assassins in his personal vendetta against the drug. He wrote in the *American Magazine* in 1937:

> In the year 1090, there was founded in Persia the religious and military order of the Assassins, whose history is one of cruelty, barbarity and murder, and for good reason. The members were confirmed users of hashish, or marijuana, and it is from the Arab "hashishin" that we have the English word "assassin." (Anslinger and Cooper, 1937)

The use of cannabis was particularly common in Egypt in the Middle Ages, where the Gardens of Cafour in Cairo became a notorious haunt of hashish smokers. Despite draconian measures by the Egyptian authorities to close such establishments and to prohibit hashish use during the thirteenth and fourteenth centuries, the habit had become too firmly ingrained in the Arab world for it to be stamped out. The social acceptance of cannabis use among the people of Egypt and other Arab lands was reinforced by the fact that while the holy Koran explicitly banned the consumption of alcohol, it did not mention cannabis. Not all were happy about this acceptance of cannabis, however. Ebn-Beitar wrote of the spread of cannabis use in Egypt 600 years ago:

> It spread insensibly for several years and became of common enough usage that in the year 1413 A.D., this wretched drug appeared publicly, it was eaten flagrantly and without furtiveness, it triumphed....One had no shame in speaking of it openly....Also as a consequence of that, baseness of sentiments and manners became general; shame and modesty disappeared among men, they no longer blushed to hold discourse on the most indecent things....And they came to the point of glorifying vices. All sentiments of nobility and virtue were lost....And all manner of vices and base inclination were displayed openly. (Walton, 1938, p. 14)

It was from Egypt that the use of cannabis as a psychoactive drug first spread to Europe and then to the Americas. When Napoleon invaded and conquered Egypt at the end of the eighteenth century, he was dismayed by what he saw as the corrupting influence of hashish on the local population and the possible debilitating effects it might have on his own soldiers, who

soon developed a liking for cannabis in this wine-free country. In 1800 one
of his generals issued a decree:

> Article 1: Throughout Egypt the use of a beverage prepared by some Mos-
> lems from hemp (hashish) as well as the smoking of the seeds of hemp, is
> prohibited. Habitual smokers and drinkers of this plant lose their reason and
> suffer from violent delirium in which they are liable to commit excesses of
> all kinds.
>
> Article 2: The preparation of hashish as a beverage is prohibited throughout
> Egypt. The doors of those cafes and restaurants where it is supplied are to be
> walled up, and their proprietors imprisoned for three months.
>
> Article 3: All bales of hashish arriving at the customs shall be confiscated and
> burnt. (Lewin, 1931)

As with all the earlier bans, this one too was largely ignored by the Egyp-
tians and Napoleon's army was soon to leave in retreat. However, the
returning French army brought back to Europe many colorful tales of
hashish and its intoxicating effects. Although cannabis had been cultivated in Europe for many centuries as a source of rope, canvas, and
other cloths and in making paper, its inebriating effects were largely
unknown—although secretly some sorcerers and witches may have included cannabis in their mysterious concoctions of drugs. In the midnineteenth century in France it became fashionable among a group of
writers, poets, and artists in Paris's Latin Quarter to experiment with
hashish. Among these was the young French author Pierre Gautier, who
became so enthused by the drug that he founded the famous Club des
Hashischins in Paris and introduced many others among the French literary world to its use. These included Alexander Dumas, Gerard de Nerval, and Victor Hugo—all of whom wrote about their experiences with
hashish. Gautier and his sophisticated literary colleagues regarded cannabis as an escape from a bourgeois environment, and described their
drug-induced experiences in flowery, romantic language. Thus, Gautier
wrote the following:

After several minutes a sense of numbness overwhelmed me. It seemed that my body had dissolved and become transparent. I saw very clearly inside me the Hashish I had eaten, in the form of an emerald which radiated millions of tiny sparks. The lashes of my eyes elongated themselves to Infinity, rolling like threads of gold on little ivory wheels, which spun about with an amazing rapidity. All around me I heard the shattering and crumbling of jewels of all colours, songs renewed themselves without ceasing, as in the play of a kaleidoscope. (Walton, 1938, p. 59)

Among the most influential of Gautier's colleagues was Charles Baudelaire, whose book *Les Paradis Artificiels* published in Paris in 1860, described the hashish experience in romantic and imaginative language:

... The senses become extraordinarily acute and fine. The eyes pierce Infinity. The ear perceives the most imperceptible in the midst of the sharpest noises. Hallucinations begin. External objects take on monstrous appearances and reveal themselves under forms hitherto unknown. They then become deformed and at last they enter into your being or rather you enter in to theirs. The most singular equivocations, the most inexplicable transpositions of ideas take place. Sounds have odour and colours are musical.

The book captured the imagination of many readers in the West and inspired further interest in the use of cannabis; it is still one of the most comprehensive and impressive accounts of the effects of cannabis on the human psyche. The use of hashish, however, did not become widespread in Europe. Cannabis use was practically unknown in Britain, for example, until the 1960s, although hemp had been cultivated for hundreds of years as a fiber and food crop. Similarly, in North America the hemp plant was imported shortly after the first settlements and was widely cultivated. Kentucky was particularly renowned for its hemp fields, and Kentucky Hemp, selected for its fiber production, is an important fiber variety. Americans seemed unaware of the peculiar properties of cannabis, and it is also unlikely that the varieties selected for hemp fiber production contained significant amounts of THC. It was not until the well-known midnineteenth-century American author Bayard Taylor wrote a lurid account of his experiences with hashish in the

Middle East that there was any awareness of the psychoactive effects of cannabis. Taylor described what happened after taking a large dose of the drug:

> The spirit (demon, shall I not rather say?) of Hasheesh had entire possession of me. I was cast upon the flood of his illusions, and drifted helplessly withersoever they might choose to bear me. The thrills which ran through my nervous system became more rapid and fierce, accompanied with sensations that steeped my whole being in inutterable rapture. I was encompassed in a seal of light, through which played the pure, harmonious colours that are born of light. . . . I inhaled the most delicious perfumes; and harmonies such as Beethoven may have heard in dreams but never wrote, floated around me." (Walton, 1938, p. 65)

Taylor's accounts were intentionally sensational and played to the nineteenth-century appetite for tales of adventure and vice in faraway places. It is unlikely that many readers were encouraged to experiment with cannabis themselves. One exception, however, was a young man called Fitz Hugh Ludlow. Ludlow experimented with many drugs, and started taking cannabis, then widely available in the United States in various pharmaceutical preparations. Ludlow's detailed accounts of his experiences and his subsequent addiction to cannabis are described in detail in his book *The Hasheesh Eater.* Ludlow was an intelligent youth of 16 when he discovered cannabis in the local drug store where he had already experimented with ether, chloroform, and opium. He used cannabis intensely for the next 3 or 4 years, and wrote of his experiences as part of his subsequent withdrawal from the drug. The book has become a classic in the cannabis literature, equivalent in importance to Baudelaire's *Les Paradis Artificiels,* and it will be referred to again in Chapter 4. Ludlow's book, however, seems to have had little impact at the time of its publication. One reviewer of his book, writing in 1857, commented that America was fortunately "in no danger of becoming a nation of hasheesh eaters."

For almost a hundred years from the midnineteenth century until 1937 cannabis enjoyed a brief vogue in Western medicine (Chapter 5). Following its introduction from Indian folk medicine, first to Britain and then to the rest of Europe and to the United States, a variety of different medicinal cannabis products were used.

The cannabis plant was introduced to Latin America and the Caribbean as early as the first half of the fifteenth century by slaves brought from Africa. It became fairly widely used in many countries in this region for its psychoactive properties, both as a recreational drug and in connection with various native Indian religious rites (Chapter 7). The term *marijuana*, a Spanish-Mexican word originally used to describe tobacco, came into general use to describe cannabis in both South and North America.

The history of marijuana use in the United States and its prohibition has been told many times (Snyder, 1971; Abel, 1943; Booth 2003). After a brief vogue in the midnineteenth century, the popularity of marijuana waned, and it was only regularly used in the United States in a few large cities by local groups of Mexicans and by African American jazz musicians. It was the wave of immigrants who entered the Southern United States from Mexico in the early decades of the twentieth century bringing marijuana with them that first brought the drug into prominence in America—and eventually led to its prohibition. It came initially to New Orleans and some other Southern cities and spread slowly in some of the major cities. There were colorful accusations that marijuana use provoked violent crime and corrupted the young. The head of the Federal Narcotics Bureau, Harry Anslinger, waged an impassioned campaign to outlaw the drug. He was the original spin doctor of his time, cleverly manipulating other government agencies, popular opinion, and the media with lurid tales of the supposed evils of cannabis. In 1937 the U.S. Congress, almost by default, passed the Marijuana Tax Act, which effectively banned any further use of the drug in medicine and outlawed it as a dangerous narcotic. Use of the drug continued to grow, however, and by the late 1930s newspapers in many large cities were filled with alarming stories about this new "killer drug."

In 1937 no less than 28 different pharmaceutical preparations were available to American physicians, ranging from pills, tablets, and syrups containing cannabis extracts to mixtures of cannabis with other drugs—including morphine, chloroform, and chloral. American pharmaceutical companies had begun to take an active interest in research on cannabis-based medicines. The hastily approved Cannabis Tax Act of 1937 put a stop to all further medical use and essentially terminated all research in the field for another 25 to 30 years. In Britain, as in many other European countries, cannabis continued to have a limited medicinal use for much longer, but this declined as more reliable new medicines became available. "Tincture of cannabis" was finally removed from the *British Pharmacopoeia* in the early 1970s, as the growing recreational use of cannabis was made illegal in the Misuse of Drugs Act of 1971.

The "demonization" of cannabis in the United States soon after its arrival from Latin America has colored attitudes to the drug ever since—not only in North America, but also worldwide. In subsequent chapters the reader can judge whether this initial reaction to cannabis was justified.

# 2

---

*The Pharmacology of Delta-9-Tetrahydrocannabinol (THC), the Psychoactive Ingredient in Cannabis*

As cannabis came into widespread use in Western medicine in the nineteenth century, it soon became apparent that the effects of plant-derived preparations were erratic. The amounts of active material that the pharmaceutical preparations contained were variable from batch to batch according to the origin of the material, the cultivation conditions, and the plant variety. Cannabis imported from India often deteriorated en route or in storage. As the chemical identity of the active ingredients was not known and there was no method of measuring them, there was no possibility of quality control. This was one of the reasons why cannabis preparations eventually fell out of favor with physicians on both sides of the Atlantic. These inadequacies, however, also motivated an active research effort to identify the active principles present in the plant preparations in the hope that the pure compound or compounds might provide more reliable medicines. The nineteenth century was a great era for plant chemistry. Many complex drug molecules, known as alkaloids, were isolated and identified from plants. Several of these were powerful poisons—for example, atropine from deadly nightshade (*Atropa belladonna*); strychnine from the bark of the tree *Nux vomica*; and muscarine from the magic mushroom, *Amanita muscaria*. Others were valuable medicines still in use today—for example, morphine isolated from the opium poppy, *Papaver somniferum*; the antimalarial drug quinine from the bark of the South American cinchona tree; and cocaine from the leaves of the coca plant. Victorian chemists were attracted by the new challenge offered by isolating the active ingredient from cannabis and attacked the problem with vigor, but initially without any notable success. Unlike the previously discovered alkaloids, which were all water-soluble organic bases that could form crystalline solids when combined with acids, the active principle of the cannabis plant proved to be almost completely insoluble in water. The active compound is in fact a viscous resin with no acidic or basic properties, so it cannot be crystallized. Since most of the previous successes of natural product chemistry had depended on the ability of chemists to extract an active drug substance from the plant with acids or alkalis and to obtain it in a pure crystalline form, it was not surprising that all of the early efforts to find the cannabis alkaloid in this way were doomed to failure. Only those who recognized that the active principle could not be extracted into aqueous solutions but required an organic solvent (usually alcohol) were able to make any real progress. T. and H. Smith, brothers who founded a pharmaceutical business in the midnineteenth century in Edinburgh based on medicinal plant extracts, described in 1846 how they extracted Indian ganja repeatedly with warm water and sodium carbonate alkali to remove the water-soluble plant materials and then extracted the remaining dried ganja residue with absolute alcohol. The alcoholic extract was treated successively with alkaline milk of lime and with sulphuric acid and then evaporated to leave a small amount of viscous resin (6% to 7% of weight of the starting material) to which they gave the name *cannabin*. It was clear from the nature of the procedures used that the resin was neither acid nor base but neutral. The purified resin proved to be highly active when tested in the then traditional manner on themselves:

> Two thirds of a grain (44 mg) of this resin acts upon ourselves as a powerful narcotic, and one grain produces complete intoxication. (Smith and Smith, 1846)

The British chemists Wood, Spivey, and Easterfield, working in Cambridge at the end of the nineteenth century, made another important advance (see review by Todd, 1946). They used Indian charas (cannabis resin) as their starting material and extracted this with a mixture of alcohol and petroleum ether. From this, by using the then new technique of fractional distillation, they isolated a variety of different materials, including a red oil or resin of high boiling point (265°C), which was toxic in animals and which they suspected to be the active ingredient; they named it *cannabinol*. A sample of the purified material was passed to the Professor of Medicine in Cambridge for further pharmacological investigation. The report published in *Lancet* in 1897 by his research assistant, Dr. C. R. Marshall (Marshall, 1897), illustrates the heroic nature of pharmacological research in that era. He described his experience on taking a sample of the material as follows:

> On the afternoon of Feb 19th last, whilst engaged in putting up an apparatus for the distillation of zinc ethyl, I took from 0.1 to 0.15 gramme of the pure substance from the end of a glass rod. It was about 2.30 P.M. The substance very gradually dissolved in my mouth; it possessed a peculiar pungent, aromatic, and slightly bitter taste, and seemed after some time to produce

a slight anaesthesia of the mucous membranes covering the tongue and fauces. I forgot all about it and went on with my work. Soon after the zinc ethyl had commenced to distil—about 3.15—I suddenly felt a peculiar dryness in the mouth, apparently due to an increased viscidity of the saliva. This was quickly followed by paraesthesia and weakness in the legs, and this in turn by diminution in mental power and a tendency to wander aimlessly about the room. I now became unable to fix my attention on anything and I had the most irresistible desire to laugh. Everything seemed so ridiculously funny; even circumstances of a serious nature were productive of mirth. When told that a connection was broken and that air* was getting into the apparatus and an explosion feared I sat upon the stool and laughed incessantly for several minutes. Even now I remember how my cheeks ached. Shortly afterwards I managed to collect myself sufficiently to aid in the experiment, but I soon lapsed again into my former state. This alternating sobriety and risibility occurred again and again, but the lucid intervals gradually grew shorter and I soon fell under the full influence of the drug. I was now in a condition of acute intoxication, my speech was slurring, and my gait ataxic. I was free from all sense of care and worry and consequently felt extremely happy. When reclining in a chair I was happy beyond description, and afterwards I was told that I constantly exclaimed, "This is lovely!" But I do not remember having any hallucinations: the happiness seemed rather to result from an absence of all external irritation. Fits of laughter still occurred; the muscles of my face being sometimes drawn to an almost painful degree. The most peculiar effect was a complete loss of time relation: time seemed to have no existence: I appeared to be living in a present without a future or a past. I was constantly taking out my watch thinking hours must have passed and only a few minutes had elapsed. This, I believe, was due to a complete loss of memory for recent events. Thus, if I walked out of the room I should return immediately, having completely forgotten that I had been there before. If I closed my eyes I forgot my surroundings and on one occasion I asked a friend standing near how he was several times within a minute. Between times I had merely closed my eyes and forgotten his existence.

*Zinc ethyl burns on contact with air and consequently must be distilled in an atmosphere of carbon dioxide. (Marshall, 1897)

Marshall's colleagues became increasingly worried about him and eventually sent for medical help, but by the time the doctor arrived at around 5:00 P.M. Marshall had begun to recover and by 6:00 P.M. he was on his way home after a cup of coffee and suffered no ill effects afterward. Despite his experience, Marshall volunteered to take another dose of the resin 3 weeks later, but this time a much smaller one (50 mg). This produced essentially the same symptoms but in a milder form. It is clear that the red oil isolated by Wood and colleagues was highly enriched in the active component or components of cannabis, and Marshall's description accurately describes the typical intoxication seen after high doses of the drug.

Although Wood and his colleagues in Cambridge had come close to purifying the active ingredient in cannabis, their further work led them down a blind alley. From the red oil they were able to isolate a crystalline material after the preparation was acetylated [which produced acetyl derivatives of any compound with a free hydroxyl (-OH) group]. After purification of this crystalline derivative and removal of the acetyl groups by hydrolysis, they succeeded in isolating a compound that they called *cannabinol* and they showed that it could apparently be extracted from various other cannabis products, including several of the cannabis-containing medicines then available. The earlier red oil fraction was now renamed *crude cannabinol.* Unfortunately, however, cannabinol was not the active ingredifent but a chemical degradation product either formed during the chemical purification procedures or present as a normal degradation product in samples of cannabis material that had been stored for too long. The findings made with the original red oil material must have been due to the presence of tetrahydrocannabinol (THC) in such samples. It was believed, erroneously, for decades after this that cannabinol was indeed the active principle of cannabis, although other laboratories were unable to repeat the findings of Wood and colleagues.

Thirty years later a brilliant young British chemist Cahn revisited the problem of cannabinol (see review by Todd, 1946). He was able to isolate the pure substance as described by Wood and colleagues, and using the improved chemical techniques available in the 1920s, he carried out a meticulous series of experiments that largely established the chemical structure of cannabinol (Fig. 2.1). Although this was not the true active principle, the new structure allowed chemists to synthesize a range of related compounds, and Cahn's work provided a great impetus to further chemistry research in this field.

At the University of Illinois in the 1940s, Roger Adams was also working on the problem (Adams, 1942). He used an alcoholic extract from which he produced red oil by distillation. From this he was able to purify a crystalline benzoic acid derivative of a compound, which he named *cannabidiol* (as it contained two hydroxyl groups), and to work out its chemical structure (Fig. 2.1). This was a real advance, as this compound—unlike the cannabinol worked on by Wood and colleagues—really is one of the naturally occurring materials in the cannabis plant. Unfortunately, though, it is not the active ingredient, and the narcotic activity that was reported by volunteers who took samples of Adams's cannabidiol must have been due to contamination with THC. Nevertheless, Adams and his group were able to synthesize various chemical derivatives of cannabidiol, including hydrogenated derivatives, the tetrahydrocannabinols, and some of these did possess potent psychoactive properties (measured both in human volunteers and

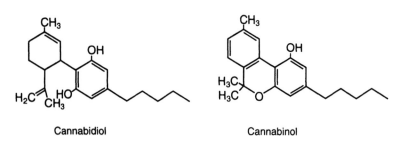

delta-9-THC                    delta-8-THC

Cannabidiol                    Cannabinol

**Figure 2.1.** Naturally occurring cannabinoids in cannabis extracts; delta-9-THC is the main psychoactive ingredient.

increasingly by observing the behavioral responses of rodents, dogs, and other laboratory animals). In his 1942 *Harvey Lecture* Adams wrote:

> The typical marijuana activity manifested by the isomeric tetrahydrocannabinols constitutes ponderable evidence that the activity of the plant itself, and of extracts prepared therefrom, is due in large part to one or other of these compounds.... (Adams, 1942)

At the same time, across the Atlantic, despite the privations of war, research on cannabinoids continued in the Chemistry Department in Cambridge England under the leadership of an outstanding organic chemist, Alexander Todd, later to become Lord Todd. He and his colleagues reisolated cannabinol and, capitalizing on the newly discovered structure of cannabidiol published by the Adams group, they were able to complete the identification of the chemical structure of this compound started by Cahn (Todd, 1946). Both the Adams group and the Todd group went on to undertake the first chemical synthesis of cannabinol, and as part of this synthesis the Cambridge team actually made delta-9-tetrahydrocannabinol as an intermediate. They commented on the high degree of biological activity that this compound possessed (assessed now by observing the characteristic behavioral reactions of dogs and rabbits rather than human subjects). The Todd group repeatedly tried to prove that this compound or something like it existed naturally in cannabis extracts. By repeated fractionation they were able to prepare a highly active and almost colorless glassy resin, which closely resembled synthetic tetrahydrocannabinol in its physical and chemical properties. The techniques available then, however, were not powerful enough to determine whether this was a single chemical substance or a complex mixture of closely related compounds. In a review article published in 1946 Todd wrote:

> ...It would appear to be established that the activity of hemp resin, in rabbits and dogs at least, is to be attributed in the main to tetrahydrocannabinols. (Todd, 1946)

THC was also isolated from a red oil fraction by the American chemist Wollner in 1942, though not as a single pure compound but as a mixture containing tetrahydrocannabinols. It was assumed for many years after the advances of the 1940s that the psychoactive properties of cannabis were due to an ill-defined mixture of such compounds. It was to be another 20 years before the brilliant chemical detective work of two Israeli scientists, Mechoulam and Gaoni, finally solved the problem and showed that in fact there is only one major active component, delta-9-THC (Fig. 2.1) (Mechoulam, 1970). Raphael Mechoulam described their introduction to this field as follows:

> When we started our then very small programme on hashish some 5–6 years ago, our interest in this fascinating field was kindled by the contrast of rich folklore and popular belief with paucity of scientific knowledge. Israel is situated in a part of the world where, for many, hashish is a way of life. Though neither a producer nor a large consumer, Israel is a crossroads for smugglers, mostly Arab Bedouin, who get Lebanese hashish from Jordan through the Negev and Sinai deserts to Egypt. Hence the police vaults are full of material waiting for a chemist. (Mechoulam, 1970)

Gaoni and Mechoulam had the advantage of new chemical separation and analytical techniques that had not been available to earlier investigators. In the Laboratory of Natural Products at the Hebrew University in Jerusalem, they had the latest methods for separating complex mixtures of chemicals by column chromatography. In this technique the mixture is poured onto a column of adsorbent material and gradually washed through by solvents. Individual compounds move down the column at different rates according to how easily they dissolve in the solvent flowing through the column. In addition, the Israeli scientists were able to employ the powerful new techniques of mass spectrometry, infrared spectroscopy, and nuclear magnetic resonance to identify the chemicals that they had separated by chromatography. In this way they were able to identify a large number of new cannabinoids in extracts of Lebanese hashish—we now know that as many as 60 different naturally occurring cannabinoids exist. Although this complexity might appear daunting, it turned out that most of the naturally occurring cannabinoids were present in relatively small amounts, or that they lacked biological activity. In fact, Gaoni and Mechoulam reported in 1964 that virtually all of the pharmacological activity in hashish extracts could be attributed to a single compound, delta-9-THC[1].

Among other chemicals in the hashish extracts Gaoni and Mechaloum identified cannabidiol (Fig. 2.1). They found a variety of other naturally occurring cannabinoids, but delta-9-THC was the most important. Cannabidiol is present in significant quantities but lacks psychoactive properties, although it may have other pharmacological effects (see below). Cannabis grown in tropical parts of the world (Africa, Southeast Asia, Brazil, Colombia, Mexico) usually has much more THC than cannabidiol, with ratios of THC/cannabidiol of 10:1 or higher. Plants grown outdoors in more northern latitudes, however (Europe, Canada, and the northern United States), usually have a much higher content of cannabidiol, often exceeding the THC content by 2:1 (Clarke, 1981, p. 159). Cannabis also contains variable amounts of carboxylic acid derivatives of delta-9-THC, and this is potentially important. Although themselves inactive, the carboxylic acid derivatives readily lose their carboxylate group as carbon dioxide on heating, which gives rise to additional active THC. This occurs, for example, when the plant material is heated during smoking or heated in the cooking processes used to form various cannabis-containing foods and drinks. This can in some instances more than double the active THC content of the original starting plant material. On the other hand, when cannabis resin or other preparations are stored, pharmacological activity is gradually lost and THC degrades by oxidation to cannabinol and other inactive materials.

The isolation and elucidation of the structure of delta-9-THC led to a burst of chemical synthetic activity around the world, as different laboratories competed to be the first to complete the synthesis of this important new natural product. The American chemists Taylor, Lenard, and Shvo were probably the first in 1967, but they were quickly followed by Gaoni and Mechoulam and by several other laboratories (for review see Mechoulam

---

1. In some publications, including those from the Israeli group, this is referred to as delta-1-tetrahydrocannabinol, but this is because there are two different conventions for numbering the chemical ring systems of which the substances are composed; the delta-9 terminology is the most commonly used.

and Hanu, 2000). The Israeli group had shown that the naturally occurring THC occurred only as the *l*-isomer, although early synthetic preparations contained a mixture of both the *l*- and *d*-optical isomers (mirror images) of the compound. So the next stage was for several laboratories to devise chemical synthetic methods that yielded only the naturally occurring *l*-isomer of delta-9-THC, which is biologically far more active than the mirror image *d*-isomer.

In retrospect, although the isolation of THC from cannabis proved technically difficult because of the nature of the compound as a neutral, water-insoluble, viscous resin, the outcome was not very different from that seen with other pharmacologically active substances derived from plants. In each case a single active compound has been identified that accounts for virtually all of the biological activity in the crude plant extracts. This active compound often exists in the plant as one member of a complex mixture of related chemicals, most of which are either minor components or lack biological activity. This is true, for example, for nicotine from the tobacco leaf, cocaine from the coca leaf, and morphine from the opium poppy.

## Man-Made Cannabinoids

The synthesis of THC was followed by a much larger synthetic chemistry effort, aimed at the discovery of more potent analogs of THC, or compounds that separated the desirable medical properties of THC from its psychoactive effects. Many hundreds of new THC derivatives were made during the 1950s and 1960s in both academic and pharmaceutical company laboratories. There were far too many to be tested on human volunteers, so most were assessed in simple animal behavior tests that had been found to predict cannabis-like activity in man (see Chapter 2). This research effort was disappointing because it proved impossible to separate the desirable properties of THC (antinausea, pain relieving) from the intoxicating effects. Nevertheless, the chemical research provided a detailed insight into the structure activity of the THC molecule—that is, which parts of the molecule are critical for psychoactivity and which parts are less important and can thus be chemically modified without losing biological activity. Several derivatives proved to be even more active than THC, working in animals and human volunteers at doses up to 100 times lower than required for THC (for review see Duane Sofia, 1978).

At the Pfizer company in the United States, for example, chemists were among the first to discover the first potent synthetic THC analog *nantradol*, which entered pilot-scale clinical trials and was found to have analgesic (pain-relieving) properties that were not blocked by the drug naloxone — an antagonist that blocks analgesics of the morphine type that act on opiate receptors. Nantradol as synthesized originally was a mixture of four chemical isomers from which the active one, *levonantradol*, was later isolated. These compounds had an important advantage over THC in being more water soluble and thus easier to formulate and deliver as a potential medicine. Further chemical work at Pfizer led to the discovery of a new chemical series of simplified THC analogs that possessed only two of the three rings of THC; among these bicyclic compounds was the potent analog CP55,940 (Fig. 2.2), which has been widely used as a valuable research compound (Table 2.1). The Pfizer compound levonantradol was tested in several clinical trials during the early 1980s. It proved to be as potent as morphine as an analgesic and was effective in blocking nausea and vomiting in patients undergoing cancer chemotherapy, but the psychoactive side effects proved to be unacceptable and the company decided to abandon further research on this project (Dr. Ken Coe, personal communication).

Work in Raphael Mechoulam's laboratory in Israel was particularly productive in generating new analogs of THC (e.g., HU-210 [Fig. 2.2], which has particularly high affinity for both CB-1 and CB-2 receptors) (Mechoulam and Hanu, 2000). Research in the pharmaceutical company Eli Lilly in the United States led to the synthesis of *nabilone* (Fig. 2.2), the only synthetic THC analog that has been developed and approved as a medicine, sold under the trade name Cesamet (Chapter 5).

In an unexpected development, research scientists at the Sterling Drug Company in the United States unwittingly discovered another chemical class of molecules that did not immediately resemble THC but

38                                THE SCIENCE OF MARIJUANA

nevertheless proved to act through the same biological mechanisms. A research program aimed at discovering novel aspirin-like anti-inflamma-
tory/pain-relieving compounds generated an unusual lead compound
called *pravadoline*. This had a remarkable profile in animal tests — it was
highly effective in a broad range of pain tests, including ones in which
aspirin-like molecules generally do not work. In addition, it failed to
cause any gastric irritation, one of the biggest drawbacks in the aspirin
class of drugs. Pravadoline also was not very effective in the key biochemical test for aspirin-like activity, the ability to inhibit the synthesis of the
inflammatory chemicals, prostaglandins. It seemed to the scientists involved that they had discovered a promising new mechanism for pain
relief — and one that might have important advantages. Pravadoline went
into clinical development, and meanwhile many other analogs were synthesized. From these emerged the compound WIN55,212-2 (Fig. 2.2)
(D'Ambra et al., 1996), an even more potent pain-relieving compound

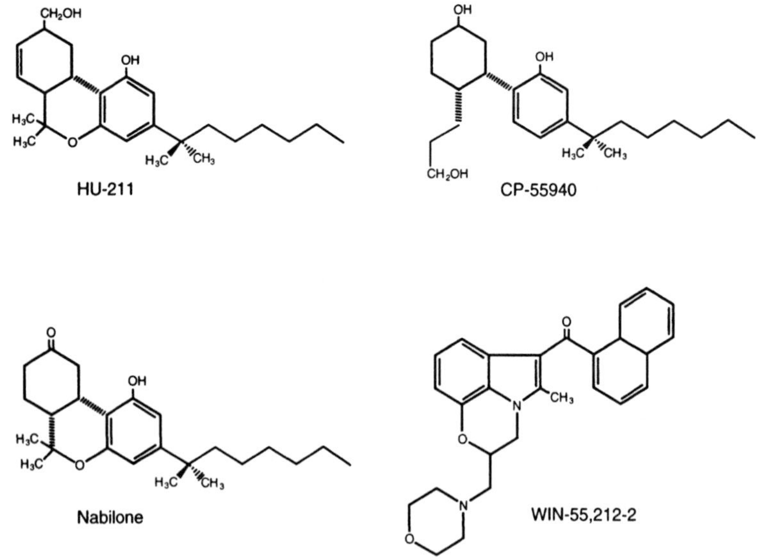

Figure 2.2. Man-made synthetic cannabinoids.

with improved absorption properties. However, when the specific receptor for cannabis was discovered in the 1980s (see below), it became clear that pravadoline and WIN55,212–2 acted like THC on this receptor (Kuster et al., 1993), and were thus pharmacologically cannabinoids rather than aspirin-like anti-inflammatory drugs. Their pain-relieving properties were not due to a new mechanism but to the same mechanism as that of cannabis. Pravadoline had by that time been tested in hum an volunteers and found to possess good effectiveness against moderate to severe pain in, for example, postoperative dental pain. But it also caused dizziness and light-headedness as an obvious limiting side effect. The development of pravadoline was dropped because of kidney toxicity, and the company then decided to abandon the whole program—partly for budget reasons and partly to avoid being associated with the image of a cannabis-like drug (Dr. Susan Ward, personal communication).

From the synthesis and testing of many hundreds of chemical analogs a consistent body of evidence was built up, which defined the chemical structure-activity rules that determine whether a molecule will be active at the CB-1 receptor (for reviews see Mechoulam and Hanu, 2000; Duane Sofia, 1978; Makriyannis and Rapaka, 1990; and Thakur et al., 2005).

## Cannabinoid Antagonists

An important recent development has been the discovery of molecules that bind to the cannabis receptor in the brain, but instead of mimicking THC, they block its actions. Like the synthetic cannabinoids, these come from various different chemical classes, and three examples are shown in Figure 2.3. The first cannabinoid antagonist to be described was the compound SR141716A, now called rimonabant, from the French pharmaceutical company Sanofi-Aventis, and this has been used extensively in the past few years both as a valuable research tool and as a new medicine for the treatment of obesity (Chapter 5). Other compounds with CB-1 antagonist activity have since been described by other pharmaceutical companies and academic laboratories (Table 2.1). Subsequently, compounds were developed that acted as selective antagonists at CB-2 receptors (e.g., SR144528).

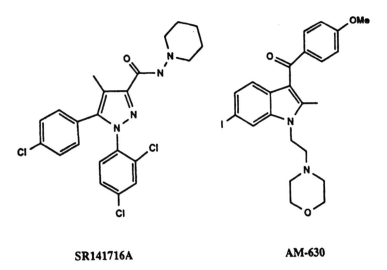

**LY320135**

**SR141716A**

**AM-630**

**Figure 2.3.** Synthetic drugs that act as antagonists at the CB-1 cannabinoid receptor. SR141716A = rimonabant (Accomplia).

Table 2.1. Cannabis Receptor (CB-1) Binding Profiles:
[H³]CP55,940 Assay of Rat Brain Membranes

| Drug | Ki—Concentration for Half Occupancy of Receptor Binding Sites—Nanomolar ($10^{-9}$ M) |
| --- | --- |
| (–)CP55,940 | 0.068 |
| (+)CP55,940 | 3.4 |
| THC | 1.6 |
| 11-hydroxy-THC | 1.6 |
| Cannabinol | 13.0 |
| Cannabidiol | >500.0 |

From Devane et al. (1988).

## How Does THC Get to the Brain?

### Smoking

Smoking is an especially effective way of delivering psychoactive drugs to the brain. When marijuana is smoked some of the THC in the burning plant material distills into a vapor (the boiling point of THC is around 200°C), and as the vapor cools the compound condenses again into fine droplets, forming a smoke, which is inhaled. As the drug dissolves readily in fats, it passes readily though the membranes lining the lungs, which offer a large surface area for absorption. The drug enters blood, which passes directly from the lungs to the heart, from where it is pumped into the arteries around the body. THC has no difficulty in penetrating the brain, and within seconds of inhaling the first puff of marijuana smoke, active drug is present on the cannabis receptors in the brain. Peak blood levels are reached at about the time that smoking is finished (Fig. 2.4).

An experienced marijuana smoker can regulate almost on a puff-by-puff basis the dose of THC delivered to the brain to achieve the desired psychological effect and to avoid overdose and minimize the undesired effects. Puff and inhalation volumes tend to be higher at the beginning and lowest at the end of smoking a cigarette (more drug is delivered in the last part of the cigarette because some THC condenses onto this). When

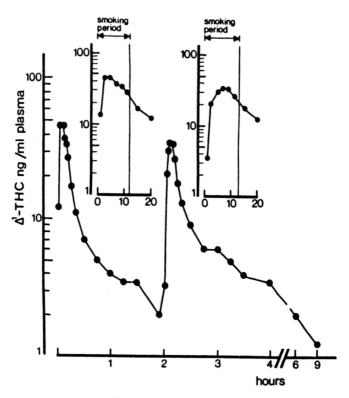

**Figure 2.4.** Average blood levels of THC in human volunteers who smoked two identical marijuana cigarettes, each containing about 9 mg of THC, 2 hours apart. Insets show the rapid absorption of the drug during the period of smoking. (From Agurell et al., 1986.)

experienced smokers were tested with marijuana cigarettes containing different amounts of THC (from 1% to 4%), without knowing which was which, they adjusted their smoking behavior to reach about the same level of THC absorption and subjective high. When smoking the less potent cigarettes puff volumes were larger and puff duration higher than with the more potent cigarettes, and when smoking the latter more air was inhaled, thereby diluting the marijuana smoke (Herning et al., 1986; Heishman et al., 1989).

Many marijuana smokers hold their breath for periods of 10 to 15 seconds after inhaling, in the belief that this maximizes the subjective response to the drug. Studies in which subjective responses and THC levels in blood were measured with different breath hold intervals, however, have failed to show that breath holding makes any real difference to the absorption of the drug—this idea thus seems to fall in the realm of folklore rather than reality.

It is clear why smoking is the preferred route of delivery of cannabis for many people. As with other psychoactive drugs, the rapidity by which smoking can deliver active drug to the brain and the accuracy with which the smoker can adjust the dose delivered are powerful pluses. The rapid delivery of drug to the receptor sites in the brain seems to be an important feature in determining the subjective experience of the high. This is true not only for cannabis, but also for other psychoactive drugs that are smoked. These include nicotine, crack cocaine, methamphetamine, and, increasingly nowadays, heroin ("chasing the dragon"). For the narcotic drugs, smoking is the only method that approaches the instant delivery of drug achieved by intravenous injection—and it does not carry the risks of infection with hepatitis or HIV associated with intravenous use. Fortunately, the extreme insolubility of cannabis precludes the use of the intravenous route.

The amount of THC absorbed by smoking, however, varies over quite a large range. Of the total amount of THC in a marijuana cigarette, on average, about 20% will be absorbed, the rest being lost by combustion, side stream smoke, and incomplete absorption in the lung. But the actual figure ranges from less than 10% to more than 30%, even among experienced smokers. (For review see Huestis, 2005.)

Oral Absorption

Taking THC by mouth is even less reliable as a method of delivering a consistent dose of the drug. THC is absorbed reasonably well from the gut, but the process is slow and unpredictable and most of the absorbed drug is rapidly degraded by metabolism in the liver before it reaches the general circulation. The peak blood levels of THC occur anywhere between 1 and 4 hours after ingestion and the overall delivery of active THC to the bloodstream averages less than 10%, with a large range between individuals.

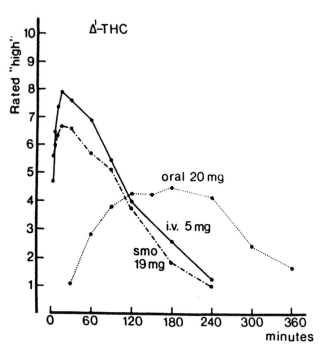

**Figure 2.5.** Time course of the subjective "high" after administering THC by different routes. Smoking gives as rapid an effect as an intravenous injection, whereas taking the drug by mouth produces a delayed and prolonged high. The subjective experience somewhat outlasts the presence of THC in blood (see Fig. 2.5) because THC persists longer in the brain. (From Agurell et al., 1986.)

The high is correspondingly also delayed by comparison with smoking (Fig. 2.5). Even for the same person the amount of drug absorbed after oral ingestion will vary according to whether he or she has eaten a meal recently and the amount of fat in his or her food. A further complication of the oral route is that one of the metabolites formed in the liver is 11-hydroxy-THC (Fig. 2.6). This is a psychoactive metabolite with potency about the same as that of THC. The amount of 11-OH-THC formed after smoking is relatively small (plasma levels are less than a third of those for THC), but

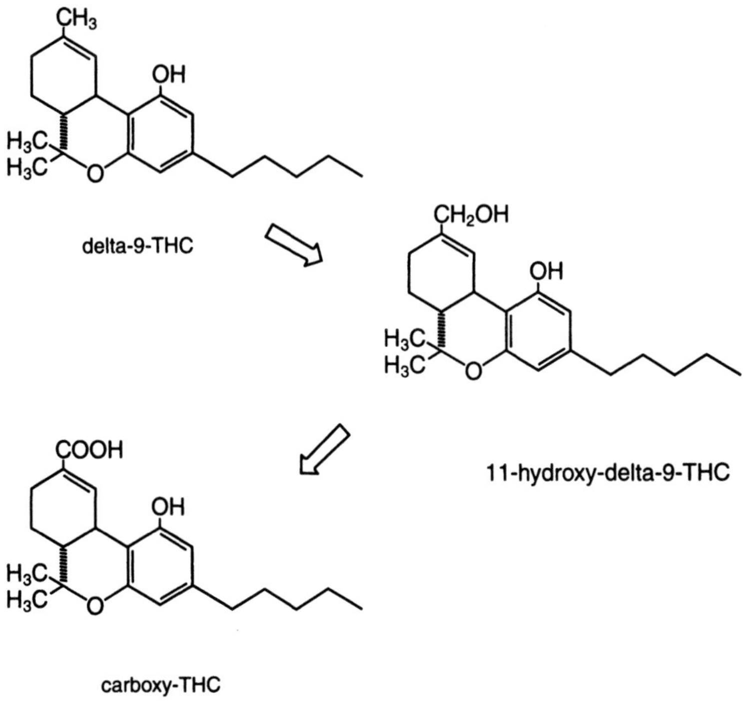

Figure 2.6. Principal route of metabolism of THC.

when cannabis is taken by the oral route—where all the blood from the intestine must first pass through the liver—the amount of 11-OH-THC in plasma is about equal to that of THC and it probably contributes at least as importantly as THC to the overall effect of the drug.

The only officially approved medicinal formulation of THC (known pharmaceutically as *dronabinol*) is in the form of capsules containing the drug dissolved in sesame oil—a product called Marinol. It is not surprising that this and other orally administered cannabis products have not proved consistently effective in their medical applications—and both patients and recreational users generally prefer smoked marijuana. The erratic and un-reliable oral absorption of THC poses a serious problem for the effective use of the pure drug as a medicine, as will be discussed again in Chapter 5.

## Other Routes of Administration

Because THC is so insoluble in water, injection by the intravenous route is very difficult. It can be achieved by slowly adding an alcoholic solution of THC to a rapid intravenous infusion of saline solution, but this is rarely used even in hospital settings. Other alternatives have been little explored so far. By dissolving THC in suitable nontoxic solvents, it is possible to deliver the drug as an inhalation aerosol to the lung, and this seems worthy of further examination. The makers of Marinol are developing a metered-dose aerosol inhalation formulation for the more rapid delivery of the drug, and this is currently in clinical trials. For more information go to http://www.medicalnewstoday.com/medicalnews.php?newsid=22937.

Another way of delivering the drug is in the form of a rectal suppository. Research on such a formulation, using a hemisuccinate ester of THC, which is gradually converted to THC, yielded promising results (El Sohly, 1996). Absorption from the rectum bypasses the liver and avoids the problem of liver metabolism, which limits the oral availability of THC, and it seems that this route can deliver about twice as much active drug to the bloodstream as the oral route, although there is still considerable variability in drug absorption from one individual to another.

Other possible delivery routes include the use of instruments designed to heat the herbal cannabis material to vaporize the THC so that it can then be inhaled (several such devices are available from Internet sites and shops specializing in cannabis accessories). The problem with this approach is that the plant material needs to be heated to close to 200°C in order to volatilize THC, but this is quite near the point of combustion, which releases noxious smoke and associated toxins. Despite this, tests of one commercially available vaporizer showed that it vaporized about half of the available THC in a sample of herbal cannabis and THC was the main component in the vapor, whereas the smoke from the conventional burning of cannabis contained more than 100 other organic compounds (Gieringer et al., 2004). It may be that vaporization will offer a safe way for the fast delivery of medical marijuana.

The only herbal cannabis product currently approved for medical use is Sativex, a standardized plant extract (Chapter 5). It is delivered by metered spray under the tongue or on the inside of the cheek. Absorption takes place fairly rapidly from the rich orobuccal blood supply. This route is used for a variety of traditional medicines (e.g., nitroglycerine) and appears to be effective.

## Elimination of THC From the Body

After smoking, blood levels rise very rapidly and then decline to around 10% of the peak values within the first hour (Fig. 2.4). The maximum subjective high is also attained rapidly and persists for about 1 to 2 hours, although some milder psychological effects last for several hours. After oral ingestion the peak for plasma THC and the subjective high are delayed and may occur anywhere from 1 to 4 hours after ingestion, with mild psychological effects persisting for up to 6 hours or more (Fig. 2.5). Although in each case unchanged THC disappears quite rapidly from the circulation, elimination of the drug from the body is in fact quite complex and takes several days. This is largely because the fat-soluble THC and some of its fat-soluble metabolites rapidly leave the blood and enter the fat tissues of the body. As the drug and its metabolites are gradually excreted in the urine (about one third) and in the feces (about two thirds), the material in the fat tissues slowly leaks back into the bloodstream and is eventually eliminated. This gives an overall elimination half-time of 3 to 5 days, and some drug metabolites may persist for several weeks after a single drug exposure (for review see Agurell et al., 1986). Urine or blood tests for one of the major metabolites, 11-nor-carboxy-THC (Fig. 2.6), use a very sensitive immunoassay and can give positive results for days or even weeks after a single drug exposure. Thus, even after a single dose of cannabis the user may test positive several days later, and regular cannabis users may remain positive for up to a month after taking the last dose. The proportion of the carboxy metabolite relative to unchanged THC increases with time and measurements of this ratio can indicate fairly accurately how long ago cannabis was consumed. What is more relevant for roadside traffic accident or workplace drug testing is an indication of recent use or intoxication, and this is better provided by the measurement of THC in samples of saliva—which

accurately reflects cannabis use within the past few hours (see http://www.
erowid.org/plants/cannabis/cannabis_testing.shtml).

The unusually long persistence of THC in the body has given cause
for some concern, but it is not unique to THC—it is seen also with a
number of other fat-soluble drugs, including some of the commonly used
psychoactive agents (e.g., diazepam [Valium]). The presence of small
amounts of THC in fat tissues has no observable effects, as the levels are
very low. There is no evidence that THC residues persist in the brain, and
the slow leakage of THC from fat tissues into blood does not give rise to
drug levels that are high enough to cause any psychological effects (figs.
2.5 and 2.6). Smoking a second marijuana cigarette a couple of hours after
the first generates virtually the same plasma levels of THC as previously
(Fig. 2.5). Nevertheless, the drug will tend to accumulate in the body if
it is used regularly. While this is not likely to be a problem for occasional
or light users, there have been few studies of chronic high-dose cannabis
users to see whether the increasing amounts of drug accumulating in fat
tissues could have harmful consequences. Is it possible, for example, that
such residual stores of drug could sometimes give rise to the "flashback"
experience that some cannabis users report—the sudden recurrence of a
subjective high not associated with drug taking?

The persistence of THC and its metabolites in the body certainly
causes confusion in other respects, particularly as drug-testing procedures can now detect very small amounts of THC and its metabolites. For
people caught with positive cannabis tests, often applied randomly in the
workplace or because they were involved in road traffic accidents or were
admitted to hospital emergency rooms, the consequences can be serious.
(For review see Huestis, 2005.)

## How Does THC Work?

### Discovery of Cannabinoid Receptors

Pharmacologists used to think that the psychoactive effects of cannabis were
somehow related to the ability of the drug to dissolve in the fat-rich membranes of nerve cells and disrupt their function. But the amount of drug

that is needed to cause intoxication is exceedingly small. An average marijuana cigarette contains 10 to 20 mg of THC (a milligram is 1/1,000 of a gram, or about 1/30,000 of an ounce). Only 10% to 20% of the total THC content is absorbed by the smoker—so an average total body dose is between 1 and 4 mg of THC. The amount of drug ending up in the brain, which accounts for only about 2% of total body weight, can be predicted to be not more than 20 to 80 µg (a microgram is 1/1,000,000 of a gram). Although these are exceedingly small amounts, they are comparable to the naturally occurring amounts of other chemical compounds used in various forms of chemical signaling in the brain. The brain works partly as an electrical machine, transmitting pulses of electrical activity along nerve fibers connecting one nerve cell to another, but the actual transmission of the signal from cell to cell involves the release of pulses of chemical signal molecules known as *neurotransmitters*. These chemicals are specifically recognized by receptors, which are specialized proteins located in the cell membranes of target cells. The neurotransmitter chemicals are released in minute quantities: for example, the total amount of one typical neurotransmitter, noradrenaline, in human brain is not more than 100 to 200 µg—a quantity comparable to the intoxicating dose of THC. This suggests that THC most likely acts by targeting one or the other of the specific chemical signaling systems in the brain, rather than by some less specific effect on nerve cell membranes, and indeed, this is what the scientific evidence suggests.

An important breakthrough in understanding the target on which THC acts in the brain was the discovery by Allyn Howlett and her colleagues at St. Louis University in 1986 of a biochemical model system in which THC and the new synthetic cannabinoid drugs WIN55,12–2 and CP55,940 were active (for reviews see Howlett, 2005; and Abood, 2005). The cannabinoids were found to inhibit the activity of an enzyme in rat brain, adenylate cyclase, which synthesizes a molecule known as cyclic adenosine monophosphate (AMP) (Fig. 2.7). The significance of this finding was that the synthesis of cyclic AMP is known to be controlled by a number of different cell surface receptors that recognize neurotransmitter substances. Some receptors, when activated, stimulate cyclic AMP formation, while others inhibit it. Cyclic AMP is known as a *second messenger*

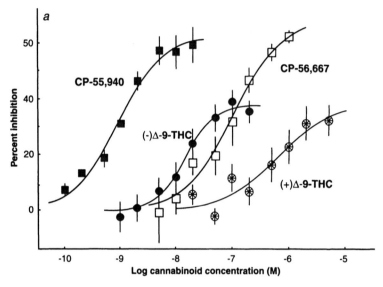

**Figure 2.7.** Inhibition of cyclic AMP formation in tissue culture cells that possess the CB-1 cannabinoid receptor. The synthetic cannabinoid CP55,940 is more potent than (–)delta-9-THC and produces a larger maximum inhibition. The response shows selectivity for the (–) isomers of the compounds versus the (+) isomers (CP56,667 is the (+) isomer of CP55,940). (From Matsuda et al., 1990.)

molecule as it is formed inside cells in response to activation of a receptor at the cell surface by some primary chemical messenger. Cyclic AMP acts as an important control molecule inside the cell, regulating many different aspects of cell metabolism and function. Thus, Howlett's discovery suggested that she had found an indirect way to study drug actions on the *cannabis receptor* in the brain. A few years later in 1988 Howlett's group went one step further and found a more direct way to study drug actions at the cannabis receptor.

A popular method for studying drug actions at cell surface receptors is to measure the selective binding of a substance known to act specifically on such a receptor to the receptor sites in fragments of brain cell membranes incubated in a test tube. In order to be able to measure the very small amounts of drug bound to the receptors—which are only present in small numbers—the drug molecule is usually tagged by incorporating a small amount of radioactivity into the molecule. The radioactive drug can then be measured very sensitively by radioactive detection equipment. Sol Snyder and his colleagues at Johns Hopkins University in Baltimore pioneered the application of this method to the study of drug receptors in the brain during the 1970s. In a now famous experiment Snyder and his student Candice Pert used a radioactively labeled derivative of morphine to show that rat brain possessed specific *opiate receptors*, which selectively bound this and all other pharmacologically active opiate drugs (Pert and Snyder, 1973). This experimental approach was subsequently used to devise binding assays for all of the known neurotransmitter receptors in the brain and peripheral tissues. Such assays offer a simple method for determining whether any compound interacts with a given receptor and provide a precise estimate of its potency by measuring what concentration is needed to displace the radiolabeled tracer.

Snyder's group and several others had tried to see whether a binding assay could be devised for the cannabis receptor by incubating rat brain membranes with radioactively labeled THC in a test tube. This failed, however, because the THC dissolves in the lipid-rich cell membranes very readily—and this nonspecific binding to the membranes completely obscured the tiny amount of radiolabeled THC bound specifically to the receptors. Howlett collaborated with research scientists at the Pfizer pharmaceutical company to solve this problem. They achieved success by using not THC, but the synthetic compound CP55,940 discovered at the company laboratory as a very potent synthetic cannabinoid (Fig. 2.2). This had the advantage of being even more potent than THC—and thus binding even more tightly to the cannabis receptor—and as CP55,940 is more water soluble than THC, there was much less nonspecific binding of the radiolabeled drug to the rat brain membrane preparations. The binding assay that resulted seemed faithfully to reflect the known pharmacology of THC and various synthetic cannabinoids (Table 2.1.) (Devane et al., 1988). Thus, THC and the psychoactive metabolite 11-hydroxy-THC were able to displace radiolabeled CP55,940 at very low concentrations—around 1 nanomolar (equivalent to less than 1 μg in a liter of fluid, compatible with the amounts of THC thought to be present in the brain after intoxicant doses). Cannabidiol and other inactive cannabinoids were inactive, and the *d*-isomer of CP55,940—known to be much less potent in animal behavior models—was some 50 times less potent in displacing the radiolabel than the more active mirror image *l*-isomer. The binding assay was quickly adopted and was used, for example, to confirm that the Sterling-Winthrop compound WIN55,212–2 acted specifically at the cannabis receptor, which most likely explained its analgesic actions. Indeed, radioactively labeled WIN55,212–2 could be used as an alternative label in binding studies to identify the cannabis receptor. Another facet of cannabis pharmacology was emphasized by the discovery of these biochemical models—namely, that the cannabis receptor seemed to be a wholly novel discovery—not related in any obvious way to any of the previously known receptors for neurotransmitters in the brain. None of the neurotransmitters themselves or the other chemical modulators in the brain, the neuropeptides, interacted to any extent in the cannabis binding assay.

The cannabis receptor in the brain belongs to a family of related receptor proteins, and in 1990 a group working at the U.S. National Institutes of Health isolated the gene encoding it (Matsuda et al., 1990). This provided independent confirmation of the unique nature of the cannabis receptor. A few years later a second gene was discovered, which encoded a similar but distinct subtype of cannabis receptor, now known as the CB-2 receptor to distinguish it from the CB-1 receptor in the brain (for review see Felder and Glass, 1998). CB-2 receptors also bind radioactively tagged CP55,940 and recognize most of the cannabinoids that act at CB-1 sites. The CB-2 receptor, however, is clearly different and is found mainly in peripheral tissues, particularly on white blood cells—the various components of the immune system of the body—although it is also present at low levels in some brain regions, notably the brainstem (Van Sickle et al., 2005). It may be that actions of THC on peripheral CB-2 sites may account for some of the effects of cannabis on the immune system. Research on the CB-2 receptors has been helped by the availability of selective antagonists at these receptors (e.g., SR 144528) and the development of $CB_2$-selective synthetic agonists (e.g., AM630, AM1241) (Pertwee, 2005b). Studies of the

## Cannabinoid Receptor: Agonists, Partial Agonists, and Inverse Agonists

Research on the cannabinoid receptor has shown that THC acts as a *partial agonist* at the CB-1 receptor; that is, it is not able to elicit the full activation of the receptor seen, for example, with the synthetic compounds CP55,940 and WIN55,212-2. This can be shown by the fact that THC does not cause the same maximum inhibition of adenylate cyclase as the synthetic compounds (Fig. 2.8). An alternative functional assay measures the ability of various agonists to stimulate the binding of a metabolically stabilized analog of guanosine triphosphate (GTP-γ-S) to the activated receptor. In this assay THC is also only partly effective (25% to 30%) by comparison with the synthetic cannabinoids. This assay also reveals some level of *constitutive* activity in the CB-1 receptor—reflected by binding of GTP-γ-S in the absence of any added cannabinoid. This is inhibited by the antagonist rimonabant, suggesting that in addition to its ability to antagonize the actions of cannabinoid agonists, this compound also acts as an *inverse agonist* at the CB-1 receptor; that is, it can block the resting level of activity in the receptor, which occurs in the absence of cannabinoid agonists. It is not clear whether such baseline receptor activity is great enough to be of any physiological significance, but if so it might explain some of the pharmacological effects that have been observed in animals when treated with the antagonist alone.

functional roles of CB-1 and CB-2 receptors have also been greatly helped by the development of genetically modified strains of mice, in which the expression of one or the other receptor has been knocked out (Valverde et al., 2005) (see Chapter 3).

It is possible that further cannabinoid receptors remain to be discovered. Groups working in the pharmaceutical industry have identified a G-protein–coupled receptor by searching DNA sequence databases. This receptor, called GPR55, is activated by THC and endocannabinoids and may be a third cannabinoid receptor, but so far most information is derived from the patent literature (Baker et al., 2006).

It is notable that the two other naturally occurring cannabinoids, cannabidiol and cannabinol, interact only weakly with either the CB-1 or CB-2 receptor. Nevertheless, these compounds in high doses do possess some pharmacological activities that do not appear to be related directly to actions on these receptors (Pertwee, 2004). Cannabidiol has been reported to possess anticonvulsant activity in some animal models of epilepsy (see Chapter 5). In some animal and human psychopharmacology experiments cannabidiol was found to possess antianxiety properties (Zuardi et al., 1982), and it has been proposed as a possible treatment for schizophrenia (Zuardi et al., 2006). The mechanisms involved are unknown, but it is possible that more cannabinoid receptors remain to be discovered (Abood, 2005).

## Neuroanatomical Distribution of CB-1 Receptors in the Brain

The distribution of cannabinoid receptors was first mapped in rat brain in autoradiographic studies, using the radioligand [$H^3$]CP55,940, which binds with high affinity to CB-1 sites. This method involves incubating thin sections of brain tissue with the radiolabeled drug and subsequently using a photographic emulsion sensitive to radiation to detect where the radiotracer was selectively bound (Herkenham et al., 1991) (Fig. 2.8). The validity of using this radioligand was confirmed by autoradiographic studies in CB-1 receptor knockout mice (genetically engineered so that they do not have any CB-1 receptors in their brains), in which no detectable [$H^3$]CP55,940 binding sites were observed (Zimmer et al., 1999). Subsequently, antibodies that target particular regions of the CB-1 receptor protein were used for immunohistochemical mapping studies (Egertová et al., 1998; Pettit et al., 1998; Egertová and Elphick, 2000). Immunohistochemistry provides a superior degree of spatial resolution than autoradiography and allows very high-resolution mapping at the electron microscope level (Mackie, 2005),

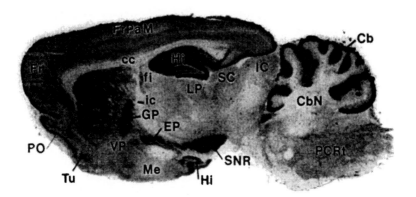

**Figure 2.8.** Distribution of cannabinoid CB-1 receptor in rat brain revealed by an autoradiograph of the binding of radioactively labeled CP55,940 to a brain section. The brain regions labeled are Cb = cerebellum; CbN = deep cerebellar nucleus; cc = corpus callosum; EP = entopeduncular nucleus; fi = fimbria hippocampus; Fr = frontal cortex; FrPaM = frontoparietal cortex motor area; GP = globus pallidus; Hi = hippocampus; IC = inferior colliculus; LP = lateral posterior thalamus; Me = medial amygdaloid nucleus; PO = primary olfactory cortex; PCRt = parvocellular reticular nucleus; SNR = substantia nigra pars reticulata; Tu = olfactory tubercle; and VP = ventroposterior thalamus. (Photograph kindly supplied by Dr. Miles Herkenham, National Institute of Mental Health, USA.)

but the overall pattern of distribution of CB-1 receptors revealed by the two approaches proved to be very similar (Elphick and Egertová, 2001; Mackie, 2005). The mapping and imaging of CB-1 receptors in the living human brain is likely to be possible soon. This will involve the use of sophisticated brain imaging technology and low doses of radiotracers that bind selectively to the receptors (Lindsey et al., 2005; Horti et al., 2006).

The mapping studies in rat brain showed that CB-1 receptors are mainly localized to axons and nerve terminals and are largely absent from the neuronal cell bodies or dendrites. The finding that cannabinoid receptors are predominantly presynaptic rather than postsynaptic is consistent with the postulated role of cannabinoids in modulating neurotransmitter release (see below). Autoradiographic mapping of CB-1 receptors in postmortem human brain revealed a very similar anatomical distribution to that seen in laboratory animals (Mackie, 2005; Lindsey et al., 2005).

In both animals and man the cerebral cortex, particularly frontal regions, contains high densities of CB-1 receptors. There are also very high densities in the basal ganglia and in the cerebellum (Fig. 2.8). In the limbic forebrain CB-1 receptors are found, particularly in the hypothalamus and in anterior cingulate cortex. The hippocampus also contains a high density of CB-1 receptors. The relative absence of the cannabinoid receptors from brainstem nuclei may account for the low toxicity of cannabinoids when given in overdose.

## Some Physiological Effects of THC

### Inhibition of Neurotransmitter Release

Although we have only a limited knowledge of how activation of the CB-1 receptor in the brain leads to the many actions of THC, some general features of cannabinoid control mechanisms are emerging. Although CB-1 receptors are often coupled with inhibition of cyclic AMP formation, this is not always the case. In some nerve cells activation of CB-1 receptors inhibits the function of calcium ion channels, particularly those of the N-subtype. This may help to explain how cannabinoids inhibit the release of neurotransmitters, since these channels are essential for the release of these substances from nerve terminals. CB-1 receptors are not usually located on the cell body regions of nerve cells—where they might control the electrical firing of the cells—but are concentrated instead on the terminals of the nerve fibers, at sites where they make contacts (known as synapses) with other nerve cells. Here the CB-1 receptors are well placed to modify the amounts of chemical neurotransmitter released from nerve terminals, and thus to modulate the process of synaptic transmission by regulating the amounts of chemical messenger molecules released when the nerve terminal is activated (see Chapter 3). Experiments with nerve cells in tissue culture or with thin slices of brain tissue incubated in the test tube have shown that the addition of THC or other cannabinoids can inhibit the stimulation-evoked release of various neurotransmitters, including the inhibitory amino acid γ-aminobutyric acid (GABA) and the amines noradrenaline and acetylcholine (Szabo and Schlicker, 2005). In the peripheral nervous system CB-1 receptors are also found on the terminals of some of the nerves that innervate various smooth muscle tissues (Mackie, 2005). Roger Pertwee and his colleagues in Aberdeen have made use of this in devising a variety of organ bath assays, in which THC and other cannabinoids inhibit the contractions of smooth muscle in the intestine, vas deferens, and urinary bladder evoked by electrical stimulation. Such bioassays have proved valuable in assessing the agonist/antagonist properties of novel cannabinoid drugs (Pertwee, 2005b).

Although cannabinoids generally inhibit neurotransmitter release, this does not mean that their overall effect is always to dampen down activity in neural circuits. For example, reducing the release of the powerful inhibitory chemical GABA would have the opposite effect, by reducing the level of inhibition. This may explain two important effects of cannabinoids that have been described in recent years: (1) that administration of THC leads to a selective increase in the release of the neurotransmitter dopamine in a region of the brain known as the nucleus accumbens and (2) that this is accompanied by an activation and increased release of naturally occurring opioids (endorphins) in the brain (see Chapter 4). (See Iversen, 2003; and Pertwee, 2005a for more detailed reviews.)

### Effects on the Heart and Blood Vessels

The cannabinoids exert quite profound effects on the vascular system. In animals, the main effect of THC and anandamide is to cause a lowering of blood pressure; in man, the effect in inexperienced users is often an increase in blood pressure, but after repeated drug use the predominant effect becomes a lowering in blood pressure. This is due to the action of THC on the smooth muscle in the arteries, causing a relaxation that leads to an increase in their diameter (vasodilation). This in turn leads to a drop in blood pressure as the resistance to blood flow is decreased, and this automatically triggers an increase in heart rate in an attempt to compensate for the fall in blood pressure. The vasodilation caused by THC in human subjects is readily seen as a reddening of the eyes caused by the dilated blood vessels in the conjunctiva. The cardiac effects can be quite large—with increases in heart rate in man that can be equivalent to as much as a 60% increase over the resting pulse rate (Fig. 2.9). Although this presents little risk to young healthy people, it could be dangerous for patients who have a history of heart disease, particularly those who have suffered a heart attack or heart failure previously. Another feature commonly seen after high doses of cannabis is *postural hypotension*; that is, people are less able to adjust their blood pressure adequately when rising from a seated or lying down position. This leads to a temporary drop in blood pressure, which in turn can cause dizziness or even fainting.

Until recently it was assumed that the effects of the cannabinoids on the heart and blood vessels were mediated indirectly through actions on receptors in the brain. It is now becoming clear, however, that many and perhaps all of these effects are mediated locally, through CB-1 receptors located in the blood vessels and heart. Isolated blood vessels relax when

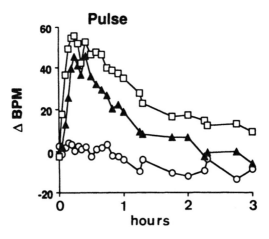

**Figure 2.9.** Effects on heart rate of smoking a single marijuana cigarette containing 1.75% THC (filled triangles) or 3.55% THC (open squares) versus placebo (open circles). Average results from six volunteer subjects studied on three separate occasions. (From Huestis et al., 1992.)

incubated with anandamide, and this effect and the vascular effects in the whole animal can be blocked by the CB-1 antagonist rimonabant. This antagonist also blocks the effects of THC on blood pressure and heart rate in animals or man. Furthermore, the cardiovascular effects of THC are completely absent in CB-1 receptor knockout mice (see Chapter 3).

Other physiological effects of cannabinoids may also be due to direct actions on CB-1 receptors on blood vessels. These include the ability to lower the pressure of fluid in the eyeball (intraocular pressure) (Pate et al., 1998)—an effect thought to be due to the presence of CB-1 receptors in small arteries in the eye—and the ability of cannabinoids to increase blood flow through the kidney, due to a direct action of the drugs on CB-1 receptors on blood vessels in the kidney. (For review see Pacher et al., 2005.)

## Effects on Pain Sensitivity

The ability of cannabinoids to reduce pain sensitivity represents an important potential medical application for these substances (see Chapter 5). THC and synthetic cannabinoids are effective in many animal models of both acute pain (e.g., mechanical pressure, chemical irritants, noxious heat) and chronic pain (e.g., inflamed joint following injection of inflammatory stimulus or sensitized limb after partial nerve damage) (Iversen and Chapman, 2002). In all these cases the pain-relieving (analgesic) effects of cannabinoids are prevented by cotreatment with the antagonist rimonabant and are absent in CB-1 receptor knockout mice, indicating that the CB-1 receptor plays a key role. In these animal models cannabinoids behave much like morphine, and THC is often found to be approximately equal in potency to morphine. CB-1 receptors are present at high densities at various relay stations in the neural pathways that transmit pain information into the central nervous system, including primary sensory pain-sensitive neurons, the spinal cord, the brainstem, and other relay sites. This distribution is similar to that of the opiate receptor and the endogenous morphine-like brain chemicals—the endorphins. But the opiate and cannabinoid systems appear to be parallel but distinct (Fields and Meng, 1997). Treatment of animals with low doses of naloxone, a highly selective antagonist of the opioid receptor, completely blocks the analgesic effects of morphine but generally has little or no effect in reducing the analgesic actions of THC or other cannabinoids. Conversely, rimonabant generally has little or no effect on morphine analgesia. Nevertheless, there are links between these two systems. In some of the animal models the analgesic effects of cannabinoids are partially prevented by treatment with naloxone. Conversely, the cannabinoid antagonist rimonabant partially blocks morphine responses in some studies. In other experiments it has been found that cannabinoids and opiates act synergistically in producing pain relief (i.e., the combination is more effective than either drug alone in a manner that is more than simply additive). For example, in the mouse tail flick response to radiant heat and in a rat model of arthritis (inflamed joint), doses of THC that by themselves were ineffective made the animals more sensitive to low doses of morphine (Smith et al., 1998). Such synergism could have potentially useful applications in the clinic (see Chapter 5).

Another interesting observation is that the CB-1 antagonist rimonabant, in addition to blocking the analgesic effects of cannabinoids, may sometimes, when given by itself, make animals more sensitive to painful stimuli—the opposite of analgesia. The simplest interpretation of this finding is that there may be a constant release of endogenous cannabinoids in pain circuits, and that these compounds thus play a physiological role in setting pain thresholds (see Chapter 3). Alternatively, some of the CB-1 receptors in the body may have some level of activation even when not stimulated by cannabinoids—rimonabant might then act as an *inverse agonist* to suppress this receptor activity.

It has generally been assumed that the site of action of the cannabinoids in producing pain relief is in the central nervous system. In support of the concept of a central site of action, several studies have shown that cannabinoids can produce pain relief in animals when they are injected directly into the spinal cord or brain. However, there is also evidence for a dual action of cannabinoids at both central nervous system (CNS) and peripheral tissue levels. In a rat inflammatory pain model, in which the irritant substance carrageenan was injected into a paw, injection of very small amounts of cannabinoids into the inflamed paw inhibited the development of increased pain sensitivity normally seen in this model. The peripheral injection of compounds selective for CB-2 receptors also caused analgesia in this model, and these effects were blocked by a CB-2–selective antagonist.

CB-2–selective agonists are also effective in a variety of pain models, and their effects are not blocked by rimonabant. It is possible that the effects of the CB-2–selective compounds are due in part to their anti-inflammatory actions in suppressing immune system responses to injury. These findings suggest an important role for peripheral sites in mediating the overall analgesic effects of cannabinoids and point to potential future applications for topically administered cannabinoids and/or CB-2–selective agonists in pain control (Walker and Hohmann, 2005). (For reviews see Iversen and Chapman, 2002; and Walker and Hohmann, 2005.)

### Effects on Motility and Posture

Cannabinoids cause a complex series of changes in animal motility and posture. At low doses there is a mixture of depressant and stimulatory effects and at higher doses predominantly CNS depression. In small laboratory animals THC and other cannabinoids cause a dose-dependent reduction in their spontaneous running activity. This may be accompanied by sudden bursts of activity in response to sensory stimuli—reflecting a hypersensitivity of reflex activity. Adams and Martin (1996) described the syndrome in mice as follows:

> $\Delta^9$-THC and other psychoactive cannabinoids in mice produce a "popcorn" effect. Groups of mice in an apparently sedate state will jump (hyperreflexia) in response to auditory or tactile stimuli. As animals fall into other animals, they resemble corn popping in a popcorn machine.

At higher doses the animals become immobile and will remain unmoving for long periods, often in unnatural postures, a phenomenon known as *catalepsy*.

Similar phenomena are observed in large animals. One of the first reports of the pharmacology of cannabis was published in the *British Medical Journal* a hundred years ago (Dixon, 1899). Dixon described the effects of extracts of Indian hemp in cats and dogs as follows:

> Animals after the administration of cannabis by the mouth show symptoms in from three quarters of an hour to an hour and a half. In the preliminary stage

cats appear uneasy, they exhibit a liking for the dark, and occasionally utter high pitched cries. Dogs are less easily influenced and the preliminary condition here is one of excitement, the animal rushing wildly about and barking vigorously. This stage passes insidiously into the second, that of intoxication....In cats the disposition is generally changed showing itself by the animals no longer demonstrating their antipathy to dogs as in the normal condition, but by rubbing up against them whilst constantly purring; similarly a dog which was inclined to be evil-tempered and savage in its normal condition, when under the influence of hemp became docile and affectionate....When standing they hold their legs widely apart and show a peculiar to and fro swaying movement quite characteristic of the condition. The gait is exceedingly awkward, the animal rolling from side to side, lifting its legs unnecessarily high in its attempts to walk, and occasionally falling. A loss of power later becomes apparent especially in the hind limbs, which seem incapable of being extended. Sudden and almost convulsive starts may occur as a result of cutaneous stimulation, or loud noises. The sensory symptoms are not so well defined, but there is a general indifference to position. Dogs placed on their feet will stay thus till forced to move by their ataxia, whilst if placed on their side they continue to lie without attempting a movement....Animals generally become more and more listless and drowsy, losing the peculiar startlings so characteristic in the earlier stage, and eventually sleep three or four hours, after which they may be quite in a normal condition.

Monkeys respond similarly to THC, with an initial period of sluggishness followed by a period of almost complete immobility. The animals typically withdraw into the far corner of the observation cage and adopt a posture that has been called the "thinker position" because the monkeys have a tendency to support their head with one hand and have a typical blank gaze. (Human marijuana users may also sometimes withdraw from contact with other members of the group and remain unmoving for considerable periods of time.)

These effects of cannabinoids most likely reflect their actions on CB-1 receptors in an area of the brain known as the basal ganglia, which is importantly involved in the control and initiation of voluntary movements, and a region at the back of the brain known as the cerebellum, which is involved in the fine-tuning of voluntary movements and the control of balance and posture. CB-1 receptors are present in some abundance in both of these brain regions (Fig. 2.9). (For review see Fernández-Ruiz and González, 2005.)

A number of authors have attempted to combine what is known of the neuroanatomical distribution of the cannabinoid system and the results of behavioral and electrophysiological studies to speculate on the neural mechanisms underlying cannabinoid modulation of psychomotor function (reviewed by Iversen, 2003). The CB-1 receptor is expressed particularly by striatal GABAergic medium-spiny projection neurons, and is abundant in regions containing the axon terminals of these cells (globus pallidus, entopeduncular nucleus, and substantia nigra reticulata, and in axon collaterals feeding back to medium-spiny projection neurons in striatum). CB-1 receptors are also abundant on the terminals of glutamatergic projection neurons from the subthalamic nucleus to the globus pallidus, entopeduncular nucleus, and substantia nigra reticulata. Cannabinoids might thus be expected to inhibit GABA release in striatum and GABA and glutamate release in the other nuclei. Sañudo-Peña et al. (1999) suggested that the primary role of the endocannabinoid system may be to inhibit tonic release of glutamate in the substantia nigra, regulating levels of basal motor activity. Exogenous cannabinoids also lead to decreased GABA release in the substantia nigra, which could lead to a disinhibition of the inhibitory nigral input to the thalamocortical pathway, resulting in inhibition of movement. To what extent the effects of cannabinoids on motor function are due to actions in the cerebellum remains unclear, although as described above it is likely that effects on posture and balance are mediated in this brain region. CB-1 receptors are known to occur abundantly on nearly all of the principal excitatory (glutamatergic) and inhibitory (GABAergic) inputs to cerebellar Purkinje cells.

The Billy Martin Tetrad

As chemical efforts to synthesize novel THC analogs and other synthetic cannabinoids intensified, it became increasingly important to have available simple animal tests that might help to predict which compounds retained THC-like CNS pharmacology—in particular, which might be

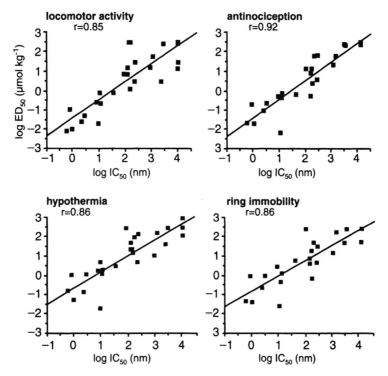

**Figure 2.10.** The Billy Martin tests. Correlation between in vivo and in vitro activities of more than 25 cannabinoid analogs to inhibit spontaneous activity ("locomotor activity"), reduce sensitivity to pain (tail-flick test) ("antinociception"), reduce body temperature ("hypothermia"), and cause immobility ("ring immobility") in mice plotted against affinities of the same compounds for CB-1 receptors assessed in an in vitro binding assay using radioactively labeled CP55,940. (Illustration from Abood and Martin, 1992.)

psychoactive in man. Although it is never possible to determine whether an animal is experiencing intoxication, certain simple tests do seem to have some predictive value. Professor Billy Martin, who is one of the leading international experts on cannabis pharmacology at the Medical College of Virginia, devised a series of four simple behavioral tests that have been widely used (Martin, 1985). He demonstrated that drugs that produced in mice a combination of reduced motility, lowered body temperature, analgesia, and immobility (catalepsy) were very likely to be psychoactive in man. The four symptoms are readily measured experimentally and exhibit dose-dependent responses to cannabinoids. By testing a large number of compounds in the *Billy Martin tetrad*, Martin and colleagues showed that there was a good correlation between the potencies of the various cannabinoids in these tests and their affinities for the CB-1 receptor, as measured in a radioligand binding assay in the test tube (Fig. 2.10). Furthermore, the CB-1 receptor antagonist rimonabant completely blocks all four responses.

# 3

*Endocannabinoids*

## Discovery of Naturally Occurring Cannabinoids—The Endocannabinoids

The existence of specific receptors for cannabinoids in the brain and in other tissues suggested that they were there for some reason. The receptors had not evolved simply to recognize a psychoactive drug derived from a plant, just as the opiate receptor was not in the brain simply to recognize morphine. In the 1970s the discovery of the opiate receptor in the brain prompted an intense search for the naturally occurring brain chemicals that might normally activate this receptor—and this revealed the existence of a family of brain peptides known as the *endorphins* (*endo*genous mor*phines*). Similarly, the discovery of the cannabis receptor prompted a search for the naturally occurring cannabinoids (now known as *endocannabinoids*) (for reviews see Mechoulam et al., 1998; Felder and Glass, 1998; Axelrod and Felder, 1998; and Di Marzo et al., 2005). These discoveries have radically changed the way in which scientists view this field of research. It has changed from a pharmacological study of how the plant-derived psychoactive drug tetrahydrocannabinol (THC) works in the brain to a much broader field of biological research on a unique natural control system, now often referred to as the *cannabinoid system*. The term *cannabinoid*, originally used to describe the 21-carbon substances found in cannabis plant extracts, is now used to define any compound that is specifically recognized by cannabinoid receptors.

Several laboratories started to work on this problem and the first endocannabinoid was discovered in Israel by Raphael Mechoulam and his colleagues, who, 30 years earlier, had first described THC as the principal active component in cannabis. The Israelis searched for naturally occurring chemicals in pig brain extracts that could displace the binding of a radioactive cannabinoid in a CB-1 receptor binding assay in the test tube, and they focused their attention on chemicals that, like THC, were soluble in fat rather than in water. They succeeded in isolating a tiny amount of a fat derivative that was active in the test tube receptor assay, and they sent some of this to the pharmacologist Roger Pertwee at the University of Aberdeen in Scotland. He had developed a simple biological assay for THC and related cannabinoids, which involved measuring their ability to inhibit the contraction of a small piece of mouse muscle in an organ bath. The newly isolated chemical was active in this test—confirming that it had THC-like biological activity. This encouraged the Israeli group to extract a larger amount of material from pig brain and to determine its chemical structure. It proved to be a derivative of the fatty acid arachidonic acid and they named it *anandamide* after the Sanskrit word *ananda* meaning bliss (Devane et al., 1992). Anandamide is a fairly simple chemical, and could readily be synthesized in larger quantities by chemists (Fig. 3.1). There have now been many studies on this endocannabinoid, which confirm that it has essentially all of the pharmacological and behavioral actions of THC in various animal models—including the "Billy Martin tetrad"— although when given to animals it is considerably less potent than THC because it is rapidly inactivated. The discovery of anandamide was not the end of the story. Mechoulam and colleagues went on to identify a second naturally occurring cannabinoid, also a derivative of arachidonic acid, known as 2-arachidonylglycerol (2-AG) (Fig. 3.1). This too was synthesized and proved to have THC-like actions in various biological tests, including whole animal behavioral models, and potency similar to that

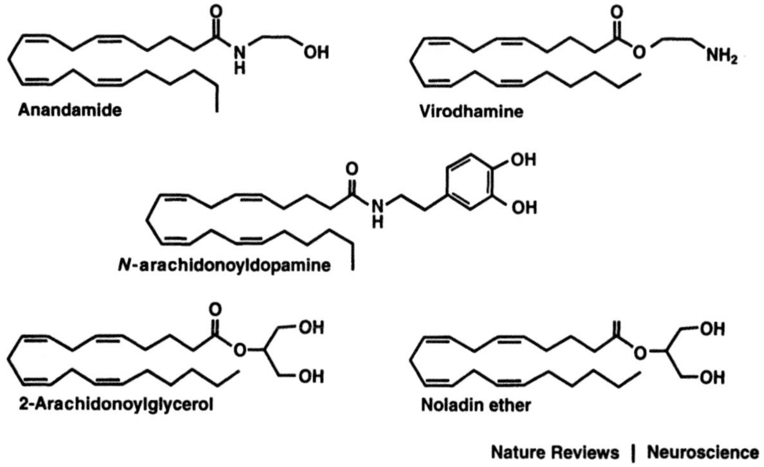

Nature Reviews | Neuroscience

Figure 3.1. Naturally occurring endocannabinoids.

of anandamide. Since then another three endocannabinoids have been described (Fig. 3.1). All are derivatives of arachidonic acid (Di Marzo et al., 2005). These compounds differ in their relative potencies at CB-1 and CB-2 receptors, with anandamide showing the most selectivity for CB-1; 2-AGE (noladin ether) and N-arachidonoyldopamine (NADA) showing some degree of CB-1 selectivity; and 2-AG being about equally potent on the two receptors. Virodhamine acts as a weak partial agonist or antagonist at the CB-1 receptor but a full agonist at the CB-2 (Porter et al., 2002). The endocannabinoids are part of a large family of other lipid signaling molecules derived from arachidonic acid, which includes the prostaglandins and leukotrienes, important mediators of inflammation. Far less is known about the newer members of the endocannabinoid group, and it remains unclear whether they all play important functional roles. The functions of the natural endocannabinoid control system are only just beginning to emerge (Piomelli, 2003; Di Marzo et al., 2005).

## Biosynthesis and Inactivation of Endocannabinoids

The endocannabinoids are derived from the unsaturated fatty acid arachidonic acid, which is one of the fatty acids found commonly in the lipids found in all cell membranes. Anandamide is synthesized by an enzyme known as phospholipase D (Di Marzo et al., 2005), but 2-AG is synthesized by a different route involving an enzyme known as diacylglycerol (DAG) lipase (Di Marzo et al., 2005). Biosynthetic routes for the other three proposed endocannabinoids remain to be elucidated. Inhibitors of the biosynthetic enzyme offer an alternative to cannabinoid receptor antagonists in dampening cannabinoid activity, and there has been some progress in discovering such inhibitors (Bisogno et al., 2006).

As with the prostaglandins and leukotrienes, the endocannabinoids are not stored in cells awaiting release, but rather are synthesized on demand. The stimulus that triggers biosynthesis is a sudden influx of calcium on activation of the cell. The rate of biosynthesis of anandamide and 2-AG in brain is increased, for example, when nerve cells are activated by exposure to the excitatory amino acid L-glutamate. Giuffrida et al. (1999) reported the first demonstration of anandamide release from the living brain using delicate microprobes inserted into rat brain. They found that anandamide release was stimulated by activation of receptors for the chemical transmitter molecule dopamine, and suggested that this might represent an automatic *dampening* system, since anandamide seemed to counteract the behavioral stimulant effects of the dopamine-like drug they used. Although 2-AG is present in larger amounts than anandamide, Giuffrida et al. (1999) found no detectable amounts of 2-AG in their release samples.

As with other biological messenger molecules, the endocannabinoids are rapidly inactivated after their formation and release. Both anandamide and 2-AG are broken down by hydrolytic enzymes. An enzyme known as *fatty acid amide hydrolase* (FAAH) seems likely to play a key role. Immunohistochemical staining of rat brain sections using antibodies against purified FAAH showed that the enzyme was most concentrated in regions containing high densities of CB-1 receptors (Ergotová et al., 1998). More detailed studies suggested that the degrading enzyme might be located particularly in those neurons that were postsynaptic to axon terminals that bore presynaptic CB-1 receptors (Elphick and Egertová, 2001). The enzyme has been cloned and sequenced; it belongs to the large family of serine hydrolytic enzymes. Rapid degradation of anandamide accounts for its relatively weak and transient actions when administered in vivo. For this reason, a number of metabolically more stable chemical analogs have been synthesized. The simple addition of a methyl group in *methanandamide*, for example, stabilizes the amide linkage and provides a molecule that retains activity at the CB-1 receptor and has greatly enhanced in vivo potency and duration (Fig. 3.2). A number of other stable analogs of both anandamide and 2-AG are available (Mechoulam et al., 1998).

After their release from cells, a specific transport protein exists to shuttle anandamide and other endocannabinoids into cells, where they can then be metabolized by FAAH. There has been some controversy about the existence of the *endocannabinoid transporter*, some arguing that the endocannabinoids simply diffuse into cells and are rapidly degraded by FAAH, which acts as a "sink," drawing them in. However, anandamide uptake appears to be real as it can still be demonstrated in the presence of inhibitors of FAAH or in FAAH knockout mice (Fegley et al., 2006). It is

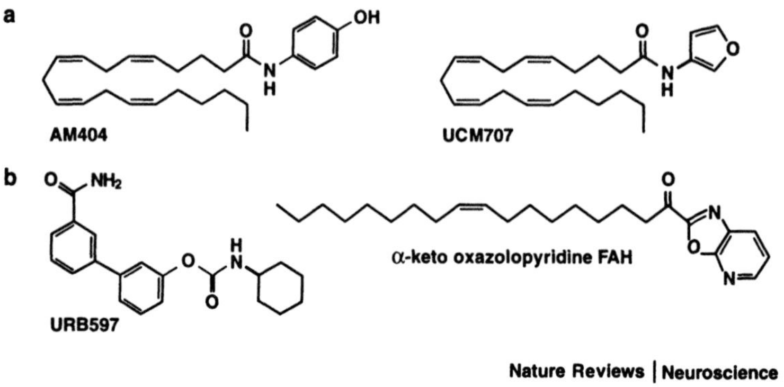

**a**

AM404

UCM707

**b**

URB597

α-keto oxazolopyridine FAH

Nature Reviews | Neuroscience

**Figure 3.2.** Examples of synthetic drugs that act as inhibitors of the endocannabinoid transporter (left) or the enzyme fatty acid amide hydrolase (right).

also possible that the transporter plays a dual role, facilitating the sudden release of anandamide and other cannabinoids from the cell when their synthesis is triggered (Di Marzo et al., 2005). Cellular uptake mechanisms are involved in the inactivation of monoamine and amino acid neurotransmitters, and these are important targets for psychoactive drug development. The antidepressant drug fluoxetine (Prozac), for example, acts by inhibiting the uptake of serotonin (5-hydroxytryptamine) and making more available to act on serotonin receptors in brain. The endocannabinoid transporter is consequently an attractive target for drug discovery (see below). (For review see Di Marzo et al., 2005.)

## Physiological Functions of Endocannabinoids

### Retrograde Signal Molecules at Synapses

Elphick and Egertová (2001) undertook immunohistochemical mapping studies of the regional distribution of CB-1 receptors and the enzyme FAAH in brain and found there was considerable overlap suggesting a complementary relationship between the two at the synaptic level. They postulated the existence of a retrograde cannabinoid signaling mechanism, whereby endogenous cannabinoids are released in response to synaptic activation, feedback to presynaptic receptors on these axon terminals, and are subsequently inactivated by FAAH after their uptake into the postsynaptic compartment. This hypothesis has been supported independently by neurophysiological findings. A phenomenon known as *depolarization-induced suppression of inhibition* (DSI) has been known to neurophysiologists for some years. It is a form of fast retrograde signaling from postsynaptic neurons back to the inhibitory cells that innervate them, suppressing inhibitory inputs for periods of up to 10 seconds or more. DSI is particularly prominent in the hippocampus and cerebellum. Wilson and Nicoll (2001) suspected that a cannabinoid mechanism might be involved. They used slice preparations of rat hippocampus and induced DSI by depolarizing neurons with minute electrical currents via microelectrodes inserted into single cells. They found that DSI was completely blocked by the CB-1 receptor antagonists AM251 or rimonabant. Wilson and Nicoll (2001) were also able to show by recording from pairs of nearby hippocampal neurons that depolarizing one of these neurons caused DSI to spread and affect adjacent neurons up to 20 μm away. The results suggested that the small, lipid-soluble, freely diffusible endocannabinoids released from single neurons can act as retrograde synaptic signals that can affect axon terminals in a sphere of influence some 40 μm in diameter. Although this is a minute volume of brain tissue, it would contain hundreds of individual neurons. Further, support for the conclusion that a cannabinoid-mediated mechanism underlies DSI came from Varma et al. (2001), who found that DSI was completely absent in hippocampal slices prepared from CB-1 receptor knockout mice. CB-1 receptors in the hippocampus are particularly abundant on the terminals of a subset of γ-aminobutyric acid (GABA)-ergic basket cell interneurons, which also contain the neuropeptide cholecystokinin (Katona et al., 1999), and these may well be the neurons involved in DSI.

Retrograde signaling by cannabinoids is not restricted to the phenomenon of DSI; subsequent research has shown it to apply to DSE (a parallel process involving suppression of excitatory inputs) and to long-term depression (LTD), an inhibitory phenomenon lasting several minutes following brief stimulation of neurons in some parts of the brain (Alger, 2006).

These findings suggest that endocannabinoids are involved in the rapid modulation of synaptic transmission in the central nervous system (CNS) by a novel retrograde signaling system causing local inhibitory effects on both excitatory and inhibitory neurotransmitter release that persist for tens of seconds or minutes. This may play an important role in the control of neural circuits, particularly in the synchronized rhythmic firing patterns of neurons in the hippocampus and elsewhere. Externally administered THC or other cannabinoids cannot mimic the physiological effects of locally released endocannabinoids because their overall effect is to cause a persistent inhibition of neurotransmitter release, not the transient effects seen with DSI and DSE. (For review see Vaughan and Christie, 2005.)

## Control of Energy Metabolism and Body Weight

Endocannabinoids play a complex role in the control of obesity and energy metabolism (Carai et al., 2006). It has long been known that cannabis users often experience sudden increases in appetite (the munchies) (see Chapter 4), and this is probably due to an action of THC on CB-1 receptors in the hypothalamus. Hypothalamic levels of endocannabinoids are raised in hungry animals and in some animal models of obesity. But the actions of cannabinoids in regulating body weight are not confined to the hypothalamic control of appetite. CB-1 receptor knockout mice are resistant to obesity induced by overfeeding—even though their food intake is markedly raised rather than reduced. CB-1 receptors in fat tissues and in the liver seem to play an important role in regulating the synthesis of fats from foodstuffs (Osei-Hyiaman et al., 2005; Bellocchio et al., 2006). The CB-1 receptor antagonist rimonabant, by blocking these peripheral and central CB-1 receptor-mediated mechanisms, may offer an important new treatment for obesity and related metabolic disorders (for details see Chapter 5).

## Regulation of Pain Sensitivity

Endocannabinoids influence sensitivity to various types of pain (for review see Walker and Hohmann, 2005). As outlined in Chapter 2, cannabinoid receptors both in the CNS and in the periphery play a role in modifying pain responsivity. This situation is complicated in the case of the endocannabinoids, as several of these compounds, notably anandamide and NADA, interact not only with cannabinoid receptors, but also with another receptor that profoundly influences pain—the vanilloid receptor TRPV-1. This is found in the sensory nerves that carry pain information into the CNS and in some parts of the brain. It is the target for capsaicin—the pungent principle of the Hungarian red pepper. Activation of the TRPV-1 protein by capsaicin causes intense pain by activating the pain-sensitive sensory nerves. Paradoxically, anandamide and NADA are also able to activate this mechanism, although not as potently or effectively as capsaicin. Nevertheless, such activation would tend to negate the analgesic effects caused by activation of CB-1 receptors on the same sensory nerves. The physiological significance of this dual action of endocannabinoids is unclear, but it may explain some of the apparently paradoxical effects of the compounds in animal models—where anandamide can sometimes increase sensitivity to pain rather than cause analgesia. It is possible that the sensitivity of the CB-1 versus TRPV-1 targets to endocannabinoids may vary according to the pathological state of the animal.

One situation in which endocannabinoids are strongly activated appears to be stress, which is known to be capable of briefly dulling pain sensitivity (the wounded soldier or football player does not feel the pain immediately). In an animal model of stress-induced analgesia, much of the effect was blocked by rimonabant, and stress led to rapid accumulations of anandamide and 2-AG in an area of brainstem (periaqueductal gray) known to play a key role in regulating pain sensitivity (Hohmann et al., 2005).

An unexpected finding is that the widely used pain killer acetaminophen (otherwise known as paracetamol or Tylenol) can be metabolized by conjugation with arachidonic acid to form the anandamide analog AM404 in the brain (Högestatt et al., 2005). AM404 is not active on CB-1 receptors, but it inhibits anandamide inactivation by tissue uptake (see below) and enhances its actions. Whether this can explain the pain-relieving properties of this popular medicine remains to be determined, but the finding that the pain-relieving properties of acetaminophen in animal models are completely blocked by rimonabant is strong evidence in favor of this idea (Bertolini et al., 2006).

Cardiovascular Control

As described in Chapter 2, CB-1 receptors are found in many blood vessels, and cannabinoids relax the smooth muscle of such vessels, causing drops in blood pressure. The endocannabinoids may achieve this in part by actions on the CB-1 receptor, partly by activation of the vanilloid TRPV-1 protein and partly by triggering release of the vasodilator nitric oxide (Randall et al., 2004; Pacher et al., 2005). But although endocannabinoids can be made by the cells lining blood vessels, they do not seem to play an important role in the basal control of blood pressure. Treatment of animals or people with the CB-1 antagonist rimonabant does not affect blood pressure, and CB-1 receptor knockout mice have normal blood pressure. However, there is evidence that endocannabinoid mechanisms may become important in pathological states such as hypertension or in mediating the sudden drops in blood pressure that occur in conditions of shock, for example, after a sudden loss of blood (Pacher et al., 2005). Other results have suggested that anti-inflammatory effects of cannabinoids acting through CB-2 receptors could help to protect against the development of atherosclerotic plaques in blood vessels—a key risk factor for heart disease (Steffens et al., 2005).

Other Functions

There are other roles for endocannabinoids: for example, in the control of human reproduction. CB-1 receptors on the fertilized blastocyst and on the cells lining the uterus help to control whether or not successful implanta- tion of the blastocyst occurs. Excessive stimulation of these CB-1 receptors can block implantation or even precipitate early abortion. Local levels of anandamide are controlled by fluctuations in the activity of the degrading enzyme FAAH that are under the control of complex hormonal and other signals, including stress. It has been suggested that drugs that were able to enhance FAAH activity might be useful in treating human infertility (Mac- carrone and Wenger, 2005).

    People take cannabis because of its pleasurable and rewarding effects (see Chapter 4). Studies of endocannabinoids and CB-1 receptor knockout mice are beginning to reveal the complex manner in which cannabinoids are involved in pleasure and reward pathways (Lupica et al., 2004; Valverde et al., 2005). CB-1 knockout mice display heightened reactions to stress, including increased fear and anxiety behavior, when exposed to novel environments or other fearful stimuli. The CB-1 knockout mice are less able to forget painful unpleasant memories. When trained to associate a tone with an electric shock they are slow to extinguish this memory when tone and shock are no longer paired (Marsicano et al., 2002). These mice also demonstrate the key role played by the CB-1 receptor in the development of dependence to THC: they do not display any of the withdrawal reactions seen in normal animals treated repeatedly with THC and then challenged with the antagonist rimonabant (see Chapter 5).

## Development of a New Endocannabinoid-Based Pharmacology

### Novel Cannabinoid Receptor Agonists or Antagonists

The discovery of multiple cannabinoid receptors and the endocannabinoids as their natural ligands offers new opportunities for the development of selective agonists or antagonists. Synthetic compounds with selectivity as agonists or antagonists for CB-2 receptors are already known, and since the CB-2 receptor is only expressed at very low levels in the CNS, the problem of unwanted CNS side effects does not exist for such compounds. However, there has been relatively little research to identify the most suitable medical applications for CB-2–selective compounds. Far more promising has been the development of antagonists with selectivity for the CB-1 receptor. One such compound, rimonabant, is already approved as a novel treatment for metabolic disorders associated with obesity, and will be reviewed in more detail in Chapter 5. (For reviews see Lambert and Fowler, 2005; Mackie, 2006; and Piomelli, 2005.)

### Inhibitors of Endocannabinoid Inactivation

There is considerable interest in the discovery and development of compounds that inhibit the inactivation of endocannabinoids via the putative endocannabinoid transporter and the enzyme FAAH. Such compounds would be expected to enhance endocannabinoid actions only in areas where there was already some activation of the cannabinoid system, making their effects far more selective and restricted than those of externally administered THC or related CB-1 receptor agonists. Early success appeared to have been achieved with the discovery of the anandamide analog AM404 (Fig. 3.2), which was unable to activate CB-1 receptors but inhibited anandamide transport in cell culture models in vitro (Beltramo et al., 1997). The compound was also active in vivo; it displayed some of the actions expected in the Billy Martin tetrad (inhibition of movement, reduced body temperature) in mice, and it was effective in reducing anxiety-like behavior (Bortolato et al., 2006) and sensitivity to pain (Costa et al., 2006). AM404 also potentiated the actions of anandamide in vitro and in vivo (Beltramo et al., 1997) and led to raised levels of anandamide in brain. A number of other inhibitors of the endocannabinoid transporter have since been reported with similar pharmacological properties, but none of these compounds are completely selective transport inhibitors; all exhibit appreciable activity also as inhibitors of the degradative enzyme FAAH, and some (notably AM404) are also capable of activating the vanilloid receptor TRPV-1 (DiMarzo et al., 2005; Ho and Hillard, 2005). The relation between the transporter and FAAH remains unclear. Fegley et al. (2004) reported that anandamide transport was relatively unaffected by inhibition of FAAH or in tissue from FAAH knockout mice, and the compound AM1172, an analog of AM404 designed to be resistant to attack by FAAH, remained active as an uptake inhibitor. But Dickson-Chesterfield et al. (2006) tested a series of compounds reported to act as inhibitors of endocannabinoid transporters and found that all the compounds had activity against both the transporter and FAAH in vitro. In cells from FAAH knockout mice, the transporter inhibitors were considerably less potent, although still active. It was concluded that there are indeed two separate protein targets, although they are closely related. Some interaction with FAAH appears to be needed to confer high potency to the uptake inhibitors.

     An alternative approach has been to develop inhibitors of the degradative enzyme FAAH. This enzyme is a member of a large family of related enzymes that degrade many different protein and amide substrates (Cravatt et al., 1996). As already indicated, the enzyme has a complementary distribution in the brain to that of the CB-1 receptor and is thought to play a key role in the inactivation of endocannabinoids after their transport into cells containing the enzyme (see above). Strong evidence in support of this was provided by studying a FAAH knockout strain of mice, which exhibited increased levels of anandamide and proved to be supersensitive to anandamide (Cravatt et al., 2001). A number of laboratories have sought to develop selective inhibitors of FAAH, not an easy task because the enzyme is quite similar to many other enzymes in the *amide hydrolase* family. Nevertheless, a number of potent and apparently selective FAAH inhibitors are now available (Fig. 3.2), and their pharmacological properties are promising. In whole animal experiments these compounds raise pain thresholds and have antianxiety properties but do not themselves cause catalepsy, lowered body temperature, or increased food intake (Mackie, 2006; Piomelli et al., 2006). FAAH inhibitors, however, may not enhance the actions of all the endocannabinoids. The existing compounds do not affect tissue levels of 2-AG, and it may be that a different enzyme, monoacylglycerol lipase, is involved in degrading this endocannabinoid (Bari et al., 2006).

These early results with inhibitors of uptake or enzymic degradation are encouraging, but it will be some time before they can be translated into new medicines. To be useful such compounds need to be absorbed when given by mouth, to penetrate readily into the brain and to have a relatively long duration of action. It may take several more years of research to attain these goals. (For reviews see Di Marzo et al., 2005; and Ho and Hillard, 2005.)

# 4

The Effects of Cannabis on the Central Nervous System

A number of approaches can be used to study the effects of drugs on the brain. We can ask people taking the drug to report their own subjective experiences—and there is a large and colorful literature of this type on marijuana. But scientists prefer to use objective methods, and there have been many experiments performed with human volunteers to determine what physiological and psychological alterations in brain function are induced by the drug. The effects that the drug has on animal behavior can also help us to understand how the drug affects the human brain. Understanding how the drug acts in the brain and which brain regions contain the highest densities of drug receptors may also provide useful clues. We can be reasonably confident that the psychic effects of cannabis are due to activation of the CB-1 receptor in brain. Huestis et al. (2001) carried out a controlled study in 63 healthy cannabis users, who received either rimonabant or placebo and smoked either a tetrahydrocannabinol (THC)-containing or placebo marijuana cigarette. The CB-1 antagonist blocked all of the acute psychological effects of the active cigarettes.

## Subjective Reports of the Marijuana High

Millions of people take marijuana because of its unique psychotropic effects. It is hard to make a precise scientific description of the state of intoxication caused by marijuana as this is clearly an intensely subjective experience not easily put into words, and the experience will vary enormously depending on many variables. Some of these are easily identified:

1. The *dose of the drug* is clearly important. It will determine whether the user merely becomes *high* (i.e., pleasantly intoxicated) or escalates to the next level of intoxication and becomes *stoned*—a state that may be associated with hallucinations and end with immobility and sleep. High doses of cannabis carry the risk of unpleasant experiences (panic attacks or even psychosis). Experienced users become adept at judging the dose of drug needed to achieve the desired level of intoxication, although this is much more difficult for naive users. The dose is also much easier to control when

the drug is smoked and more difficult to control when taken by mouth.

2. The subjective experience will depend heavily on the environment in which the drug is taken. The experience of drug taking in the company of friends in pleasant surroundings is likely to be completely different from that elicited by the same dose of the drug administered to volunteer subjects studied under laboratory conditions or, as in some of the earlier American studies, to convicts in prison who had "volunteered" as experimental subjects.

3. The drug experience will also depend on the mood and personality of the user, his or her familiarity with cannabis, and his or her expectations of the drug. The same person may experience entirely different responses to the drug depending on whether he or she is depressed or elated beforehand. Familiarity with the drug means that the user knows what to expect, whereas the inexperienced user may find some of the elements of the drug experience unfamiliar and frightening. The person using the drug for medical reasons has entirely different expectations from those of the recreational user, and he or she commonly finds the intoxicating effects of cannabis disquieting and unpleasant.

There are many detailed descriptions of the marijuana experience in the literature; among the best known are the flowery and often lurid literary accounts of the nineteenth-century French authors Baudelaire, Gautier, and Dumas and those written by the nineteenth-century Americans Taylor and Ludlow. Ludlow's book, *The Hasheesh Eater*, published in 1857, gives one of the best accounts, and will be quoted frequently. Fitz Hugh Ludlow was an intelligent young man who experimented with various mind-altering drugs. He first encountered marijuana at the age of 16 in the local pharmacy, and became fascinated by the drug and eventually addicted to it. His book vividly describes the cannabis experience, although it is worth bearing in mind that he regularly consumed doses of herbal cannabis extract that would be considered very large by current standards—probably equivalent to several cannabis cigarettes in one session. In modern times there have been several surveys of the experiences of marijuana users. Among these the books by E. Goode (1970), *The Marijuana Smokers*, and by J. Berke and C. H. Hernton (1974), *The Cannabis Experience*, which review the 1960s and 1970s experiences of young American and British cannabis users, respectively, are particularly useful. For "trip reports" from contemporary marijuana users, go to http://www.lycaeum.org/drugs/trip.report.

The various stages of the experience can be separated into the *buzz* leading to the *high* and then the *stoned* states, and finally the *come-down*. The buzz is a transient stage, which may arrive fairly quickly when smoking. It is a tingling sensation felt in the body, in the head, and often in the arms and legs, accompanied by a feeling of dizziness or lightheadedness.

> With hashish a "buzz" is caused, i.e. a tingling sensation forms in the head and spreads through the neck and across the shoulders. With a very powerful joint this sensation is sometimes "echoed" in the legs.
>
> Usually the first puff doesn't affect me, but the second brings a slight feeling of dizziness and I get a real "buzz" on the third. By this I mean a sudden wave of something akin to dizziness hits me. It's difficult to describe. The best idea I can give is to say that for a moment the whole room, people, and sounds around me recede into the distance and I feel as I my mind contracted for an instant. When it has passed I feel "normal" but a bit "airy-fairy." (Berke and Hernton, 1974)

During the initial phase of intoxication the user will often experience bodily sensations of warmth (caused by the drug-induced relaxation of blood vessels and increased blood flow, for example, to the skin). The increase in heart rate caused by the drug may also be perceived as a pounding pulse. Marijuana smokers also commonly feel a dryness of the mouth and throat and may become very thirsty. This may be exacerbated by the irritant effects of marijuana smoke, but is also experienced when the drug is taken by mouth.

The influence of the drug on the mind is far-reaching and varied; the marijuana high is a very complex experience. It is only possible to highlight some of the common features here. THC has profound effects on the highest centers in the brain and alters both the manner in which sensory inputs are normally processed and analyzed and the thinking process itself. Mental and physical excitement and stimulation usually accompany the initial stages of the "high." The drug is a powerful euphoriant, as described so well by Ludlow. Some hours after taking an extract of cannabis he was:

> ...smitten by the hashish thrill as by a thunderbolt. Though I had felt it but once in life before, its sign was as unmistakable as the most familiar thing of daily life.... The nearest resemblance to the feeling is that contained in our idea of the instantaneous separation of soul and body.

The hashish high was experienced while Ludlow was walking with a friend, and the effects could be felt during the walk and after they returned home.

> The road along which we walked began slowly to lengthen. The hill over which it disappeared, at the distance of half a mile from me, soon became to be perceived as the boundary of the continent itself.... My awakened perceptions drank in this beauty until all sense of fear was banished, and every vein ran flooded with the very wine of delight. Mystery enwrapped me still, but it was the mystery of one who walks in Paradise for the first time.... I had no remembrance of having taken hasheesh. The past was the property of another life, and I supposed that all the world was revelling in the same ecstasy as myself. I cast off all restraint; I leaped into the air; I clapped my hands and shouted for joy.... I glowed like a new-born soul. The well known landscape lost all of its familiarity, and I was setting out upon a journey of years through heavenly territories, which it had been the longing of my previous lifetime to behold.... In my present state of enlarged perception, time had no kaleidoscope for me; nothing grew faint, nothing shifted, nothing changed except my ecstasy, which heightened through interminable degrees to behold the same rose-radiance lighting us up along our immense journey.... I went on my way quietly until we again began to be surrounded by the houses of the town. Here the phenomenon of the dual existence once more presented itself. One part of me awoke, while the other continued in perfect hallucination. The awakened portion felt the necessity of keeping in side street on the way home, lest some untimely burst of ecstasy should startle more frequented thoroughfares.

The nineteenth-century physician H. C. Wood of Philadelphia described his experimental use of cannabis extract:

> It was not a sensuous feeling, in the ordinary meaning of the term. It did not come from without; it was not connected with any passion or sense. It was simply a feeling of inner joyousness; the heart seemed buoyant beyond all trouble; the whole system felt as though all sense of fatigue were forever banished; the mind gladly ran riot, free constantly to leap from one idea to another, apparently unbound from its ordinary laws. I was disposed to laugh; to make comic gestures. (Walton, 1938, p. 88)

The initial stages of intoxication are accompanied by a quickening of mental associations and this is reflected typically by a sharpened sense of humor. The most ordinary objects or ideas can become the subjects of fun and amusement, often accompanied by uncontrollable giggling or laughter.

> I often feel very giggly, jokes become even funnier, people's faces become funny and I can laugh with someone else who's stoned just by looking at them.

> I would start telling long involved jokes, but would burst out laughing before completion.

> I nearly always start laughing when in company and have on numerous occasions been helpless with laughter for up to half-an-hour non-stop. (Berke and Hernton, 1974)

This effect of the drug is hard to explain, as we know so little about the brain mechanisms involved. Humor and laughter seem to be unique human features. A sharpened sense of humor and increased propensity to laugh are not unique to THC; they are seen with other intoxicants—notably with alcohol. A visit to any lively pub in Britain will confirm this phenomenon. However, THC does seem to be remarkably powerful in inducing a state that has been described as *fatuous euphoria*.

As the level of intoxication progresses from *high* to *stoned* (if the dose is sufficiently large), users report feeling relaxed, peaceful, and calm; their senses are heightened and often distorted; they may have apparently profound thoughts and they experience a curious change in their subjective sense of time. As in a dream, the user feels that far more time has passed than in reality it has. As E. Goode puts it:

Somehow, the drug is attributed with the power to crowd more 'seeming' activity into a short period of time. Often nothing will appear to be happening to the outside observer, aside from a few individuals slowly smoking marijuana, staring into space and, occasionally, giggling at nothing in particular, yet each mind will be crowded with past or imagined events and emotions, and significance of massive proportions will be attributed to the scene, so that activity will be imagined where there is none. Each minute will be imputed with greater significance; a great deal will be thought to have occurred in a short space of time. More time will be conceived of as having taken place. Time, therefore, will be seen as being more drawn out. (Goode, 1970)

Young British cannabis users report similar experiences:

The strongest feeling I get when I am most stoned is a very confused sense of time. I can start walking across the room and become blank until reaching the other side, and when I think back it seems to have taken hours. Many records seem to last much longer than they should.

Perhaps the 'oddest' experience is the confusion of time. One could walk for five minutes and get hung up on something and think that it is an hour later or the other way around, i.e. watch a movie and think it only took five minutes instead of two hours. (Berke and Hernton, 1974)

Research work at Stanford University in the 1970s by Frederick Melges and colleagues on cannabis users led him to conclude that the disorientation of time sense might represent a key action of the drug, from which many other effects flowed (Melges et al., 1971). His subjects tended to focus on the present to the exclusion of the past or future. Not having a sense of past or future could lead to the sense of depersonalization that many users experience. Focus on the present might also account for a sense of heightened perception, by isolating current experiences from those in the past. This loss of the normal sense of time is probably related to the rush of ideas and sensations experienced during the marijuana high. The user will become unable to maintain a continuous train of thought, and no longer able to hold a conversation.

> Sometimes I find it difficult to speak simply because I have so many thoughts on so many different things that I can't get it all out at once. (Berke and Hernton, 1974)

Perception becomes more sensitive, and the user has a heightened appreciation of everyday experiences. A nurse describes seeing the Chinese-style pagoda in Kew Gardens in London under the influence of marijuana:

> It was like the pagoda had been painted a bright red since I had last seen it— about an hour before. The colour was not just bright, but more than bright, it was a different hue altogether, a deep red, with lots of added pigments, a red that was redder than red. It was a red that leapt out at you, that scintillated and pulsated amid the grey sky of a typical dull English afternoon. Never in a thousand years will I forget that sight. It was like my eyes had opened to colour for the first time. And ever since then, I have been able to appreciate colour more deeply. (Berke and Hernton, 1974)

New insight and appreciation of works of art have often been reported. Many users report that their appreciation and enjoyment of music is especially enhanced while high; they gain the ability to comprehend the structure of a piece of music, the phrasing, tonalities, and harmonies and the way that they interact. Some musicians believe that their performance is enhanced by marijuana, and this undoubtedly accounted for the popularity of marijuana among jazz players in the United States in the early years of the century. Ludlow described his experience of attending a concert while under the influence of the drug:

> A most singular phenomenon occurred while I was intently listening to the orchestra. Singular, because it seems one of the most striking illustrations I have ever known of the preternatural activity of sense in the hasheesh state, and in an analytic direction. Seated side by side in the middle of the orchestra played two violinists. That they were playing the same part was obvious from their perfect uniformity in bowing; their bows, through the whole piece,

rose and fell simultaneously, keeping exactly parallel. A chorus of wind and stringed instruments pealed on both sides of them, and the symphony was as perfect as possible; yet, amid all that harmonious blending, I was able to detect which note came from one violin and which from the other as distinctly as if the violinists had been playing at the distance of a hundred feet apart, and with no other instruments discoursing near them.

While there is no evidence that cannabis is an aphrodisiac, it may enhance the pleasure of sex for some people because of their heightened sensitivity and loss of inhibitions. But if the user is not in the mood for sex, getting high by itself will not alter that:

Hash increases desire when desire is already there, but doesn't create desire out of nothing. (Berke and Hernton, 1974)

The increased sensitivity to visual inputs tends to make marijuana users favor dimly lit rooms or dark sunshades, as they find bright light unpleasant. The mechanisms in the brain that modulate and filter sensory inputs and set the level of sensitivity clearly become disinhibited. The analysis of sensory inputs by the cerebral cortex also changes, in some ways becoming freer ranging and in other ways becoming less efficient. For example, as intoxication becomes more intense, sensory modalities may overlap, so that, for example, sounds are seen as colors, and colors contain music, a phenomenon psychologists refer to as *synesthesia*.

I have experienced synesthesia—I "saw" the music from an Indian sitar LP. It came in the form of whirling mosaic patterns. I could change the colours at will. At one time a usual facet of a high was that musical sound would take on a transparent crystal, cathedral, spatial quality. (Berke and Hernton, 1974)

The peak of intoxication may be associated with hallucinations (i.e., seeing and hearing things that are not there). Cannabis does not induce the powerful visual hallucinations that characterize the drug lysergic acid diethylamide (LSD), but fleeting hallucinations can occur, usually in the visual domain.

...occasionally hallucinations. I will see someone who is not there, the much described 'insects' which flutter around at the edge of vision, patterns move and swirl. (Berke and Hernton, 1974)

At the most intense period of the intoxication the user finds difficulty in interacting with others and tends to withdraw into an introspective state. Thoughts tend to dwell on metaphysical or philosophical topics and the user may experience apparently transcendental insights:

> For a single instant, one telling and triumphant moment, I pierced what Blake might have called "the Mundane Shell." I saw shapes swimming in a field of neon bands, surging with the colors of Africa. I saw the world before my eyes through the alchemical crystal revealed, at once, in its simultaneous complexity and simplicity. My third eye must have blinked. But only a glimpse—and then, a ripple, a slackening of intensity, and the moment was lost.... This was the most intense visionary experience I have ever had. And all from a humble green vegetable." (http://www.lycaeum.org/drug/trip. report) September 7, 1998

The peak period of intoxication is also commonly associated with daydreams and fantasies.

> Fantasies, your thoughts seem to run along on their own to the extent that you can relax and 'watch' them (rather like an intense day-dream).... Images come to mind that may be funny, curious, interesting in a story-telling sort of way, or sometimes horrific (according to mood). Also many other variations. (Berke and Hernton, 1974)

The nature of the fantasies varies according to personality and mood. One of the most common fantasies is that of power. The user feels that he or she is a god, that he or she is indestructible, and that all his or her desires can be satisfied immediately. Not surprisingly, people find such fantasy states enjoyable and cite them as one of the reasons for their continued use of the drug. Ludlow described it as follows:

> My powers became superhuman; my knowledge covered the universe; my scope of sight was infinite.... All strange things in mind, which had before

been my perplexity, were explained—all vexed questions solved. The springs of suffering and of joy, the action of the human will, memory, every complex fact of being, stood forth before me in a clarity of revealing which would have been the sublimity of happiness.

A curious feature of the cannabis high is that its intensity may vary intermittently during the period of intoxication, with periods of lucidity intervening. There is often the strange feeling of *double consciousness*. Subjects speak of watching themselves undergo the drug-induced delirium, of being conscious of the condition of their intoxication yet being unable or unwilling to return to a state of normality. Experienced users can train themselves to act normally and may even go to work while intoxicated.

As the effects of the drug gradually wear off there is the *coming down* phase. This may be preceded by a sudden feeling of hunger (munchies), often associated with feelings of emptiness in the stomach. There is a particular craving for sweet foods and drinks, and an enhanced appreciation and enjoyment of food.

When I am coming down I generally feel listless and physically weak.... Often the high ends with a feeling of tiredness, this can be overcome, but is usually succumbed to when possible if not by sleep, by a long lay down.... Conversation initially becomes lively and more intense but as the high wears off and everyone becomes sleepy it usually stops. (Berke and Hernton, 1974)

The cannabis high is often followed by sleep, sometimes with colorful dreams.

However, the cannabis experience is not always pleasant. Inexperienced users in particular may experience unpleasant physical reactions. Nausea is not uncommon, and may be accompanied by vomiting, dizziness, and headache. As users become more experienced they learn to anticipate the wave of lightheadedness and dizziness that are part of the buzz. Even regular users will sometimes have very unpleasant experiences, particularly if they take a larger dose of drug than normal. The reaction is one of intense fear and anxiety, with symptoms resembling those of a panic attack, and sometimes accompanied by physical signs of pallor (the so-called *whitey*), sweating, and shortness of breath. The psychic distress can be intense, as described by young British users:

> I once had what is known as "the horrors" when I had not been smoking long. The marijuana was a very strong variety, far stronger than anything I had ever smoked before, and I was in an extremely tense and unhappy personal situation. I lost all sense of time and place and had slight hallucinations — the walls came and went, objects and sounds were unreal and people looked like monsters. It was hard to breathe and I thought I was going to die and that no one would care.
>
> I have felt mentally ill twice when using hashish. On both occasions I felt that I could control no thoughts whatsoever that passed through my mind. It was as though my brain had burst and was distributed around the room. I knew that a short time beforehand I had been quite sane, but that now I was insane and I was desperate because I thought that I would never reach normality again. I saw myself in the mirror, and although I knew that it, the person I saw was me, she appeared to be a complete stranger, and I realized that this was how others must see me. Then the head became estranged from the body — flat piece of cardboard floating a few inches above the shoulders. I was completely horrified, but fascinated, and stood and watched for what must have been some minutes. (Berke and Hernton, 1974)

As is so often the case, Ludlow's description of a cannabis-induced horror is particularly graphic. After he had taken a much larger dose of cannabis than usual — in the mistaken belief that the preparation was weaker than the one he had used most recently — he went to sleep in a dark room:

> ...I awoke suddenly to find myself in a realm of the most perfect clarity of view, yet terrible with an infinitude of demoniac shadows. Perhaps, I thought, I am still dreaming; but no effort could arouse me from my vision, and I realized that I was wide awake. Yet it was an awaking which, for torture, had no parallel in all the stupendous domain of sleeping incubus. Beside my bed in the centre of the room stood a bier, from whose corners drooped the folds of a heavy pall; outstretched upon it lay in state a most fearful corpse, whose livid face was distorted with the pangs of assassination.

The traces of a great agony were frozen into fixedness in the tense position of every muscle, and the nails of the dead man's fingers pierced his palms with the desperate clinch of one who has yielded not without agonizing resistance....I pressed my hands upon my eyeballs till they ached, in intensity of desire to shut out this spectacle; I buried my head in the pillow, that I might not hear that awful laugh of diabolic sarcasm....The stony eyes stared up into my own, and again the maddening peal of fiendish laughter rang close beside my ear. Now I was touched upon all sides by the walls of the terrible press; there came a heavy crush, and I felt all sense blotted out in the darkness.

I awaked at last; the corpse had gone, but I had taken his place upon the bier. In the same attitude which he had kept I lay motionless, conscious, although in darkness, that I wore upon my face the counterpart of his look of agony. The room had grown into a gigantic hall, whose roof was framed of iron arches; the pavement, the walls, the cornice were all of iron. The spiritual essence of the metal seemed to be a combination of cruelty and despair....I suffered from the vision of that iron as from the presence of a giant assassin.

But my senses opened slowly to the perception of still worse presences. By my side there gradually emerged from the sulphurous twilight which bathed the room the most horrible form which the soul could look upon unshattered—a fiend also of iron, white hot and dazzling with the glory of the nether penetralia. A face that was the ferreous incarnation of all imaginations of malice and irony looked on me with a glare, withering from its intense heat, but still more from the unconceived degree of inner wickedness which it symbolized....Beside him another demon, his very twin, was rocking a tremendous cradle framed of bars of iron like all things else, and candescent with as fierce a heat as the fiends.

And now, in a chant of the most terrible blasphemy which it is possible to imagine, or rather of blasphemy so fearful that no human thought has ever conceived it, both the demons broke forth, until I grew intensely wicked merely by hearing it....Suddenly the nearest fiend, snatching up a pitchfork (also of white hot iron), thrust it into my writhing side, and hurled me shrieking into the fiery cradle.

After more terrible visions Ludlow eventually cried out for help and a friend brought him water and a lamp, upon which his terrors ceased. He was to experience both "superhuman joy and superhuman misery" from the drug, but became dependent upon it and took it for many years, until after a long struggle he finally gave it up.

## Laboratory Studies of Marijuana in Human Volunteers

The sudden popularity of marijuana use among young people in 1960s America prompted an upsurge of scientific research on the drug's effects. A large and often confusing literature emerged, partly because the topic was politically charged from the outset and bias undoubtedly colored some of the investigations. Some researchers seem to have been intent on proving that marijuana was a harmful drug. Others tended to emphasize the benign aspects of the drug.

Studying a psychotropic drug under laboratory conditions is never easy. It is difficult, for example, to ensure that subjects receive a standard dose because of the inconsistent absorption of THC—even by regular users. Many of the early studies in the United States used illicit supplies of marijuana of dubious and inconsistent potency. Standardized marijuana cigarettes eventually became available for academic research studies. They were produced for the National Institute on Drug Abuse, using cannabis plants grown for the government agency by the University of Mississippi. When methods became available for measuring the THC content of the plant material, it was possible by judicious blending of marijuana of high and low THC content to produce marijuana cigarettes with a consistent THC content. By using plant material with low THC content or marijuana from which THC had been extracted by soaking in alcohol, *placebo* cigarettes with little or no THC could also be produced.

The question of how to select suitable human subjects for such studies is also difficult. The effects of marijuana in inexperienced or completely naive subjects taking it for the first time are very different from those seen in experienced regular drug users. In one of the very first controlled studies, carried out at Boston University, drug-naive subjects were compared with experienced users. As in many subsequent studies, the naive users showed larger drug-induced deficits in the various tasks designed to test cognitive and motor functions than drug-experienced subjects, who often show no deficits at all (Weil et al., 1968).

## Effects on Movement and Driving

Animal experiments have shown that THC has characteristic effects on the ability to maintain normal balance; movements become clumsy and at higher doses the animals maintain abnormal postures and may remain immobile for considerable periods (Adams and Martin, 1996). Marijuana similarly affects human subjects, impairing their performance in tests of balance and reducing their performance in tests that require fine psychomotor control (e.g., tracking a moving point of light on a screen with a stylus) or manual dexterity (for review see Iversen, 2003). There is a tendency to slower reaction times, although this is a relatively small effect and some studies failed to observe it. In these respects marijuana has similar effects to those observed with intoxicating does of alcohol. An obvious concern is whether these impairments make it unsafe for marijuana users to drive while intoxicated. Driving not only requires a series of motor skills, but also involves a complex series of perceptual and cognitive functions. There have been numerous studies in which the effects of marijuana have been assessed on performance in driving simulators and even a few studies that were conducted in city traffic. Much to everyone's surprise, the results of many of these studies revealed only relatively small impairments in driving skills, even after quite large doses of the drug. Several of the early studies showed no impairments at all, but as the driving simulators grew more sophisticated and the tasks became more complex and demanding, impairments were observed, for example, in peripheral vision and lane control. Marijuana users, however, seem to be aware that their driving skills may be impaired and they tend to compensate by driving more slowly, keeping some distance away from the vehicle ahead and in general taking fewer risks (Smiley, 1986). This is in marked contrast to the effects of alcohol, which produces clear impairments in many aspects of driving skill as assessed in driving simulators. Alcohol also tends to encourage people to take greater risks and to drive more aggressively. There is no question that alcohol is a major contributory factor to road traffic accidents; it is implicated in as many as half of all fatal road traffic accidents. Nevertheless, driving while under the influence of marijuana cannot be recommended as safe. Studies in North America and Europe have found that as many as 10% of the drivers involved in fatal accidents tested positive for THC. However, in a majority of these cases (70% to 90%) alcohol was detected as well. It may be that the greatest risk of marijuana in this context is to amplify the impairments caused by alcohol when, as often happens, both drugs are taken together (Robbe, 1998). Investigators in Canada (Bédard et al., 2007) reviewed drug and alcohol data from U.S. drivers aged 20 to 49 who were involved in a fatal crash from 1993 to 2003 and sought to determine whether drivers who tested positive for cannabis but negative for alcohol were more likely to have engaged in risky driving behavior than drivers who tested negative for both cannabis and alcohol. They concluded that the 1,647 alcohol-free drivers who tested positive for cannabis had a 29% excess risk of having driven in a fashion that may have contributed to the crash, compared to drivers who tested negative for cannabis. But motorists who had a blood alcohol content of 0.05%, a threshold well below the legal limit for drunk driving in the United States, had a 101% excessive risk of having driven in a risky manner compared to alcohol-free drivers, and drivers with a blood alcohol content of 0.10%, just over the U.S. legal limit for drunk driving, had a 200% excess risk.

### Higher Brain Function, Including Learning and Memory

There have been numerous studies of higher brain functions in human subjects given intoxicating doses of marijuana. The results did not always confirm the subjective experiences of the subjects. Thus, while subjectively users report a heightened sensitivity to auditory and visual stimuli, laboratory tests failed to reveal any changes in their sensory thresholds. If anything, they become less sensitive to auditory stimuli. The feeling of heightened sensitivity must, therefore, involve higher perceptual processing centers in the brain, rather than the sensory systems themselves. On the other hand, the perceived changes in the sense of time are readily confirmed by laboratory studies. Subjects were asked to indicate when a specified interval of time had passed or to estimate the duration of an interval of time generated by the investigator; in such tests intoxicated subjects overestimated the amount of elapsed time (Matthew et al., 1998). Thus, marijuana makes people experience time as passing more quickly than it really is; in other words, marijuana increases the subjective time rate. One minute seems like several. This curious effect can also be seen in rats trained to respond for food reward using a fixed interval schedule. When treated with THC or WIN55,212–2, the animals shortened their response interval, whereas the antagonist rimonabant lengthened this interval (Han and Robinson, 2001).

Many studies have looked for impairments in mental functioning and memory (Earleywine, 2002). In simple mental arithmetic tasks or repetitive visual or auditory tasks, which require the subject to remain attentive and vigilant, marijuana seems to have little effect on performance, although if the task requires the subject to maintain concentration over prolonged periods of time (>30 minutes), performance falls off. By far the most consistent and clearcut acute effect of marijuana is to disrupt short-term memory. Short-term memory is nowadays usually described as *working memory*. It refers to the system in the brain that is responsible for the short-term maintenance of information needed for the performance of complex tasks that demand planning, comprehension, and reasoning. As described by Baddeley (1996), working memory has three main components: a "central executive" and two subsidiary short-term memory systems, one concerned with auditory and speech-based information and the other with visuospatial information. These systems hold information on line and monitor it for possible future use. Working memory can be tested in many ways. In the expanded digit-span test subjects are asked to repeat increasingly longer strings of random numbers both in the order in which they are presented and backwards. In this test marijuana has been reported to produce a dose-dependent impairment in most studies. Other tests involve the presentation of lists of words or other items and subjects are asked to recall the list after a delay of varying interval. Again, people intoxicated with marijuana show impairments, and as in the digit-span tests they characteristically exhibit intrusion errors; that is, they tend to add items to the list that were not there originally. The drug-induced deficits in these tests become even more marked if subjects are exposed to distracting stimuli during the delay interval between presentation and recall. Marijuana makes it difficult for subjects to retain information on line in working memory in order to process it in any complex manner. This is consistent with the results of brain imaging studies, which showed that changes in blood flow 60 minutes after THC administration to volunteers were greatest in the frontal cortex, and this is where there was the best correlation with subjective reports of intoxication (Matthew et al., 1997). The frontal cortex contains the highest densities of CB-1 receptors of all cortical regions (Herkenham et al., 1991) and is known to be important in the control of executive brain function: coordinating information in short-term stores and using it to make decisions or to begin to lay down more stable memories. The hippocampus, another region enriched in cannabinoid receptors, interacts importantly with the cerebral cortex, particularly in visuospatial memory and in the processes by which working memory can be converted to longer term storage.

While marijuana has profound effects on working memory, it has little or no effect on the ability to recall accurately previously learned material—it thus seems to have no effect on well-established memories. The relatively severe impairment of working memory may help to explain why during the marijuana high subjects have difficulty in maintaining a coherent train of thought or in maintaining a coherent conversation—they simply cannot remember where the train of thought or the conversation began or the order of the components required to make sense of the information. (For reviews see Earleywine, 2002; and Riedel and Davies, 2005.)

## Comparisons of Marijuana With Alcohol

Alcohol and marijuana are both drugs usually taken in a social context for recreational purposes. Alcohol could be described as the intoxicant for the older generation and marijuana that for the young, although both drugs are quite often consumed together. How do they compare in their effects on the brain? In many ways they are quite similar. A number of studies performed under laboratory conditions have reported that users actually find it difficult to distinguish between the immediate subjective effects of acute intoxication with the two drugs.

Like marijuana, alcohol causes psychomotor impairments, a loss of balance, and a feeling of dizziness or light-headedness. In terms of cognitive performance, both drugs cause impairments in short-term memory while leaving the recall of long-term memories intact. But there are obviously some notable differences. Interestingly, the sense of time perception in subjects intoxicated with alcohol is changed in the opposite direction to that observed with marijuana. Tests similar to those described for marijuana above reveal that whereas marijuana speeds up the internal clock, alcohol slows it down—1 minute may seem like an infinity to the marijuana user but feels like only 30 seconds to the alcohol user. Whereas marijuana tends to make users relaxed and tranquil, alcohol may release aggressive and violent behavior. In terms of the long-term effects of chronic use, alcohol has none of the subtlety of marijuana. Heavy long-term use can lead to organic brain damage and psychosis or dementia (a condition known as Korsakoff syndrome), while even moderately heavy use can lead to quite severe persistent intellectual impairment.

## What Can Animal Behavior Experiments Tell Us?

Studying the actions of psychotropic drugs in animals is inherently difficult—the animals cannot tell us what they are experiencing. The application of ingenious behavioral tests, however, can tell us a great deal about how a drug "feels" to an animal. One technique that is widely used assesses the discriminative stimulus effects of CNS drugs. In this test the animals, usually rats, are trained to press a lever in their cage in order to obtain a food reward, usually a small, attractively flavored food pellet, and the reward is given automatically after a certain number of lever presses. The animals are then presented with two alternative levers and must learn to press one (the saline lever) if they had received a saline injection just before the test session or the other (the drug lever) if they had been injected with the active test drug. Pressing the wrong lever provides no food reward. In other words, the animal is being asked, "How do you feel? Can you tell that you just received a psychoactive drug?" Animals are tested every day for several weeks, receiving drug or saline randomly, and they gradually learn to discriminate the active drug from the placebo (saline). They are judged to have learned the discrimination if they successfully gain a food reward with a minimal number of presses of the wrong lever.

This technique has provided a great deal of valuable information about cannabis and related drugs. Rats and monkeys successfully recognize THC or various synthetic cannabinoids within 2 to 3 weeks of daily training (Fig. 4.1). The doses of cannabinoids that animals recognize are quite small—less than 1 mg/kg orally for THC, and much less for the

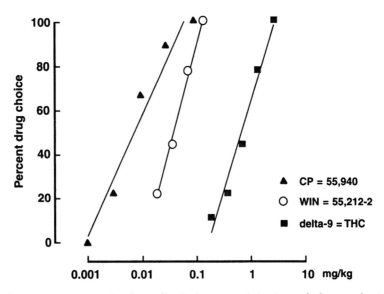

Figure 4.1. Rats trained to discriminate an injection of the synthetic cannabinoid WIN55,212–2 (0.3 mg/kg, given subcutaneously) from saline also recognize lower doses of this compound and the other psychoactive cannabinoids CP55,940 (given subcutaneously) and THC (given orally). Graph shows percentage of animals selecting the "drug" lever after various doses of the cannabinoids. Results from a group of nine rats. (From Pério et al., 1996.)

synthetic cannabinoids WIN55,212-2 and CP55,940 given subcutaneously (0.032 mg/kg and 0.007 mg/kg, respectively) (Fig. 4.1) (Pério et al.,
1996; Torbjörn et al., 1974; Wiley et al., 1995). These doses are in the
range known to cause intoxication in human subjects. When animals
have been trained to discriminate one of these drugs, the experimenter
can substitute a second or third drug and ask the animal another question: "Can you tell the difference between this drug and the one you were
previously trained to recognize?" The results of such experiments show
that rats and monkeys trained to recognize one of the cannabinoids will
generalize (i.e., judge to be the same) to any of the others. They will not
generalize, however, to a variety of other CNS-active drugs, including
psilocybin, morphine, benzodiazepines, and phencyclidine, suggesting
that cannabinoids produce a unique spectrum of CNS effects that the
animal can recognize. In all of these studies it was found that rimonabant
completely blocked the effects of the cannabinoids; that is, when animals
are treated with the cannabinoid together with the antagonist, they are
no longer able to recognize the cannabinoid. These results, thus, provide
further strong support for the hypothesis that the CNS effects of THC and
other cannabinoids are directly attributable to their actions on the CB-1
receptor in the brain.

Using these techniques, one can also ask whether the endogenous cannabinoid anandamide really mimics THC and the other cannabinoids. Rats
trained to recognize a synthetic cannabinoid do generalize to anandamide,
but high doses of anandamide are needed as it is rapidly inactivated in the
body. Monkeys do not generalize to anandamide, probably because it is inactivated too quickly. However, if monkeys are given a synthetic derivative
of anandamide that is protected against metabolic inactivation, then they
will generalize to this.

In another study rats were trained to recognize THC and were then
exposed to cannabis resin smoke. They recognized the cannabis smoke as
though it were THC and showed full generalization. In the same study
it was found that delta-9-THC and delta-8-THC were recognized interchangeably, but there was no generalization between cannabinol or cannabidiol and either THC or cannabis smoke. These results support the
hypothesis that THC is the major psychoactive component in cannabis

resin and suggest that cannabinol and cannabidiol have little psychoactive effects.

There is a large literature on the effects of THC and other cannabinoids on various aspects of animal behavior. Unfortunately, many studies have used very high doses of THC and the results consequently may have little relevance to how the drug affects the human brain. The human intoxicant dose for THC is less than 0.1 mg/kg, but doses several hundred times higher than this have often been used in animal studies. Such high doses of THC depress most aspects of animal behavior and may cause catalepsy and eventually sleep. Work with much smaller doses of cannabinoids has shown the importance of using the appropriate dose. De Fonseca and colleagues (1997) found that low doses of the synthetic cannabinoid HU-210 (0.004 mg/kg) produced behavioral effects in rats suggestive of an antianxiety effect. The test they used was to place the animals in an unfamiliar, brightly lit, large open test space containing a dark box to which the animals could retreat. Untreated animals confronted with this novel and unknown environment tended to spend much of their time in the dark box. The animals treated with HU-210, however, appeared to be less fearful and spent more of their time exploring the new environment. If the dose of HU-210 was increased to 0.02 or 0.1 mg/kg, a completely different result was obtained: the animals behaved as though they were more anxious, and spent most of their time in the dark box. In addition, the levels of the stress hormone corticosterone were increased in their blood, suggesting that the high-dose cannabinoid had activated a stress reaction. These findings may have their counterpart in the human experience that low doses of marijuana tend to relieve tension and anxiety, whereas larger doses can sometimes provoke an unpleasant feeling of heightened anxiety or even a panic reaction.

In another study the same group found that administration of low doses of rimonabant induces anxiety-like effects in the rat, using the same fear-of-novelty type of behavioral tests (Navarro et al., 1997). These findings are very intriguing: they suggest that endogenous cannabinoids in the brain may play a role in fear and anxiety responses and that there is some tonic level of activation of CB-1 receptors in the brain by these compounds that can be blocked by rimonabant.

Given the prominent impairment of working memory induced by marijuana in human subjects, it is not surprising that cannabinoids also impair working memory in animals, although there seem to have been rather few such studies. In animals there are a number of ways of assessing working memory. One model frequently used in rodents to assess spatial working memory is the radial maze. In this, a rat or mouse is placed at the center of a maze with eight arms projecting away from the central area. At the start of each experiment all eight arms will contain a food reward. To begin, the animal is placed at the center of the maze and enters one arm to retrieve a food reward. The animal is then returned to the central area and all eight arms are temporarily blocked by sliding doors. After a delay, usually of only a few seconds, the doors are opened again and the animal is free to retrieve more food rewards. Success depends on being able to remember which arms had already been visited, to avoid fruitless quests. After daily training for 2 to 3 weeks, the animals became quite expert at the task and retrieved all eight food rewards while making few errors. THC and other cannabinoids will disrupt the behavior of such trained animals in a dose-dependent manner. Furthermore, this effect of the cannabinoids can be prevented by rimonabant, showing that it is due to an action of THC on CB-1 receptors. The synthetic cannabinoids CP55,940 and WIN55,212–2 are also effective in this model and they are considerably more potent than THC. CP55,940 will also disrupt this behavior when injected in minute amounts directly into the rat hippocampus, a structure known to be particularly important for spatial memory.

Another behavioral test of memory that can be employed both in rodents and in monkeys is the delayed matching to sample task. When using this test in monkeys an animal is confronted with a number of alternative panels on a touch screen. At the start of the experiment one of these panels is illuminated and the screen then goes dead, preventing the animal from making any immediate response. After a delay, usually of 30 to 90 seconds, all the panels on the screen are illuminated and the animal has to remember which one was illuminated earlier and press it to obtain a food reward. After daily training sessions animals become proficient at this spatial memory task and make few errors. THC and other cannabinoids

again disrupt behavior in these tests of working memory. Similar results
have been observed in rats using a variant of this task.

The results of a recent study suggest the possibility that the ongoing
release of endogenous cannabinoids in the brain may play a role in modulating memory processes; the study employed an unusual memory task,
which involves a social recognition. When adult rats or mice are exposed
for the first time to a juvenile animal, they spend some time contacting
and investigating it. If the adult is exposed to the same juvenile within an
hour of the first encounter, it appears to recognize that it has already encountered this juvenile and will spend less time investigating it. If the delay
between trials is increased to 2 hours, however, the adult seems to have
largely forgotten the original encounter and investigates the juvenile animal thoroughly once more. This short-term memory appears to rely mainly
on olfactory cues. Researchers at the Sanofi Company in France found
that animals treated with low doses to the antagonist rimonabant showed
improved memory function in this test, and were able to retain the social
recognition cues for 2 hours or more. They also showed that the performance of aged rats, who had difficulty in remembering for even as long as
45 minutes, could be significantly improved by treatment with the antagonist drug (Terranova et al., 1996). This raises the intriguing possibility that
cannabinoid receptor antagonists could possibly have beneficial effects in
elderly patients who suffer from memory loss. The powerful effects of the
cannabinoid drugs in the test may be related to the fact that social recognition in rodents importantly involves olfactory cues, and the CB-1 receptor
is present in especially high densities in the olfactory regions of the brain.

The cellular basis of these effects of cannabis on higher brain function
remains unclear. Cannabinoids have been shown to disrupt the phenomenon of *long-term potentiation* in the hippocampus (Riedel and Davies,
2005). In this model, slices of rat hippocampus are incubated in saline and
electrical activity recorded from nerve cells by miniature electrodes. A burst
of electrical stimulation to the input nerve pathways to the hippocampus
leads to a long-lasting potentiation of synaptic transmission in this circuit,
so that further periods of less intense stimulation lead to greater responses
than previously. This form of plasticity in neural circuits is thought to be
critical in the laying down of memory circuits in the brain.

## Does Repeated Use of Marijuana Lead to Tolerance and Dependence?

Many drugs when given repeatedly tend to become less effective so that larger doses have to be given to achieve the same effect; that is, *tolerance* develops. There are many examples of tolerance to THC and other cannabinoids in animals treated repeatedly with these drugs. Tolerance can be seen even after treatment with quite modest doses of THC, but is most profound when large doses (>5 mg/kg) are employed. With very high doses (as much as 20 mg/kg/day), animals may become almost completely insensitive to further treatment with THC. When animals become tolerant to THC they also demonstrate cross-tolerance to any of the other cannabinoids, including the synthetic compounds WIN55,212–2 and CP55,940. This suggests that the mechanism underlying the development of tolerance has something to do with the sensitivity of the cannabinoid receptors or some mechanism downstream of these receptors, rather than simply to a more rapid metabolism or elimination of the THC. Repeated treatment with THC in both animals and people does tend to lead to an increased rate of metabolism of the drug—probably because drug-metabolizing enzymes in the liver are induced by repeated exposure to the drug. But these changes are not big enough to explain the much larger changes in sensitivity seen in responses to the drug—these include effects on cardiovascular system, body temperature, and behavioral responses. A more likely explanation is that repeated exposure to high doses of THC leads to a compensatory decrease in the sensitivity or number of cannabinoid receptors in brain. Several studies have reported decreases in the density of CB-1 receptor binding sites in the brains of rats treated for 2 weeks with high doses of THC or CP55,940 (reviewed by Lichtman and Martin, 2005).

In human volunteers exposed repeatedly to large doses of THC under laboratory conditions, tolerance to the cardiovascular and psychic effects can be produced as in the animal studies. However, it is not clear that tolerance occurs to any significant extent in people who use modest amounts of marijuana (Earleywine, 2002). The casual user, taking the drug infrequently, or those using small amounts for medical purposes seem to develop little if any tolerance. Patients in clinical trials of a cannabis-based medicine maintained a constant dose for periods of more than 1 year (Chapter 5). Tolerance seems only likely to become important for heavy users who are taking gram quantities of resin on a daily basis.

This question of whether regular users become dependent on the drug has proved to be one of the most contentious in the whole field of cannabis research. Those opposed to the use of marijuana believe that it is a dangerous drug of addiction, by which young people can easily become hooked. On the other hand, proponents of cannabis claim that it does not cause addiction and dependence at all, and users can stop at any time of their own free will. To understand these opposing views, it is important to be clear what we mean when we use the terms *tolerance, addiction,* and *dependence.* As the House of Lords report (1998) puts it:

> The consumption of any psychotropic drug, legal or illegal, can be thought of as comprising three stages: use, abuse and addiction. Each stage is marked by higher levels of drug use and increasingly serious consequences.
>
> Abuse and addiction have been defined and redefined by various organisations over the years. The most influential current system of diagnosis is that published by the American Psychiatric Association (DSM-IV, 1994). This uses the term "substance dependence" instead of "addiction," and defines this as a cluster of symptoms indicating that the individual continues to use the substance despite significant substance-related problems. The symptoms may include "tolerance" (the need to take larger and larger doses of the substance to achieve the desired effect), and "physical dependence" (an altered physical state induced by the substance which produces physical "withdrawal symptoms," such as nausea, vomiting, seizures and headache, when substance use is terminated); but neither of these is necessary or sufficient for the diagnosis of substance dependence. Using DSM-IV, dependence can be defined in some instances entirely in terms of "psychological dependence"; this differs from earlier thinking on these concepts, which tended to equate addiction with physical dependence.

For details, see the DSM-IV Criteria for Substance Dependence box.

## DSM-IV Criteria for Substance Dependence (American Psychiatric Association, 1994)

A maladaptive pattern of substance abuse, leading to clinically significant impairment or distress, as manifested by three (or more) of the following, occurring at any time in the same 12-month period:

(1) Tolerance, as defined by either of the following:
    (a) A need for markedly increased amount of the substance to achieve intoxication or desired effect
    (b) Markedly diminished effect with continued use of the same amount of the substance
(2) Withdrawal, as defined by either of the following:
    (a) The characteristic withdrawal syndrome for the substance
    (b) The same (or a closely related) substance is taken to relieve or avoid withdrawal symptoms
(3) The substance is often taken in larger amounts or over a longer period than was intended.
(4) There is a persistent desire or unsuccessful efforts to cut down or control substance use.
(5) A great deal of time is spent in activities necessary to obtain the substance (e.g., visiting multiple doctors or driving long distances), use the substance (e.g., chain-smoking), or recover from its effects.
(6) Important social, occupational, or recreational activities are given up or reduced because of substance use.
(7) The substance use is continued despite knowledge of having a persistent or recurrent physical or psychological

problem that is likely to have been caused or exacerbated by
the substance (e.g., current cocaine use despite recognition
of cocaine-induced depression or continued drinking despite
recognition that an ulcer was made worse by alcohol consumption).

Substance abuse with physiological dependence is diagnosed if
there is evidence of tolerance or withdrawal.
Substance abuse without physiological dependence is diagnosed if there is no evidence of tolerance or withdrawal.

This way of thinking about drug dependence is significantly different
from much of the earlier work in this field. It means that neither tolerance nor physical dependence need necessarily be present to make the
diagnosis of substance dependence. This has particularly changed the way
in which cannabis is viewed nowadays. It has often been argued that since
neither tolerance nor physical dependence is a prominent feature of regular marijuana users, the drug cannot be addictive. The DSM-IV definition
of substance dependence is made as the result of a carefully structured in-
terview, and the diagnosis rests on the presence or absence of various items
from a checklist of symptoms. When such assessments are made on groups
of regular marijuana users, a surprisingly high proportion is diagnosed
as dependent; these findings will be discussed in more detail in Chapter 7.

There have also been developments in basic animal research that
point to similarities between cannabis and other drugs of addiction. The
availability of rimonabant, for example, has shown that physical dependence accompanied by a withdrawal syndrome can be seen in animals that
have been treated for some time repeatedly with THC or other cannabinoid when they are challenged with the antagonist drug. The withdrawal
signs in rats included "wet dog shakes" (a characteristic convulsive shaking of the body as though the animal's fur was wet—a behavior also seen
typically during opiate withdrawal); scratching and rubbing of the face;

compulsive grooming; arched back; head shakes; spasms; and backward walking. In dogs, the withdrawal signs included withdrawal from human contact; restlessness; shaking and trembling; vomiting; diarrhea; and excess salivation. The reason why such withdrawal signs are not normally seen in animals or in people when cannabinoid administration is suddenly stopped is probably related to the long half-life of THC and some of its active metabolites in the body. This means that the CB-1 receptor is still exposed to low levels of cannabinoid for some time after the drug is stopped. With the antagonist drug, however, the CB-1 receptor is suddenly blocked. It used to be thought that cessation of cannabis use was not associated with withdrawal in human users, but carefully controlled studies have shown that a reliable and clinically significant withdrawal syndrome does occur. The symptoms include craving for cannabis, decreased appetite, sleep difficulty, and weight loss, and the syndrome may sometimes be accompanied by anger, aggression, increased irritability, restlessness, and strange dreams (Budney et al., 2001).

The animal findings with a rimonabant challenge have an interesting parallel with research on the benzodiazepine tranquilizers, of which Valium (diazepam) is the best known example. These too were thought not to be addictive, since there was little evidence for any withdrawal syndrome on terminating drug treatment. When the first benzodiazepine receptor antagonist drug flumazenil became available, though, it soon became clear that withdrawal signs could be precipitated in drug-treated animals when challenged with this antagonist. As with THC, the benzodiazepines persist for long periods in the body so drug withdrawal can never be abrupt. It is now generally recognized that benzodiazepine tranquilizers and sleeping pills do carry a significant risk of dependence with repeated use.

One way in which scientists can assess the addictive potential of psychoactive drugs is to see whether animals can be trained to self-administer them. Self-administration of heroin or cocaine is easily learned by rats, mice, and monkeys. Indeed, rats will self-administer cocaine to the exclusion of all other behavior, including feeding and sex. They have to be given restricted access to the drug to avoid damaging their health. It has proved much more difficult or impossible to train animals to self-administer THC, however, and this has often been used to argue that THC has no addictive liability. But THC is very difficult to administer to animals because of its extreme insolubility, which precludes intravenous injection, the preferred route for giving addictive drugs. Mice, however, readily learn to self-administer the more potent and water-soluble cannabinoid WIN55,2212–2 (Ledent et al., 1999).

Another series of experiments in animals has revealed that in common with other drugs of addiction, THC is able to selectively activate nerve cells in the brain that contain the chemical transmitter dopamine. French et al. (1997) in Arizona first reported that small doses of THC activated the electrical discharge of dopamine-containing nerve cells in the ventral tegmentum region of rat brain—which they recorded electrically with microelectrodes. Tanda et al. (1997) subsequently confirmed this by direct measurements of dopamine release from the nucleus accumbens region of the rat brain, which contains the terminals of the nerves originating from the ventral tegmentum (Fig. 4.2). They perfected a delicate technique that involves the insertion of minute probes into this region of rat brain, through which chemicals released in the brain can be monitored continuously in conscious, freely moving animals (a method known as microdialysis). Earlier work from this group and a number of other laboratories had shown that a number of drugs of addiction selectively activate dopamine release in this region of the brain; the drugs included heroin, cocaine, d-amphetamine, and nicotine. To this list they added THC, adding to speculation about its status as a drug of addiction. Furthermore, the Italian group reported that the THC-induced release of dopamine seemed to involve an opioid mechanism—since the effect of THC could be prevented by treatment of the animals with naloxonazine, a drug that potently and selectively blocks opioid receptor sites in brain. These results thus suggested that THC acts in part by promoting the release of opioid peptides in certain regions of the brain, and that one of the consequences of this is to cause an increase in dopamine release in the nucleus accumbens. The precise biological meaning of this remains unclear. Most scientists do not believe that dopamine release per se explains the pleasurable effects of drugs of addiction—but it does seem to have some relation to whether the animal or person will seek to obtain further doses of

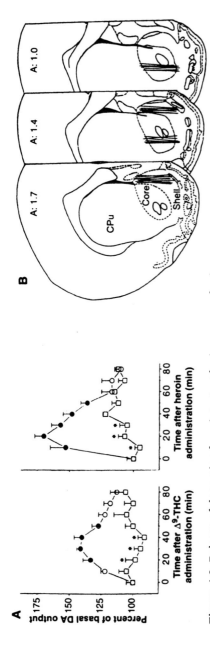

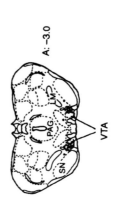

Figure 4.2. Release of dopamine from intact rat brain measured using microdialysis probes. A: Dopamine release is stimulated by the administration of THC (0.15 mg/kg, i.v.) or heroin (0.03 mg/kg, i.v.) (circles). Filled circles indicate data points that were significantly different from baseline control values. In animals treated with the opiate m receptor antagonist naloxonazine, neither THC nor heroin any longer caused dopamine release (squares). B: Sections of rat brain drawn to indicate the positions of the microdialysis probes in the individual animals used. Core = core of nucleus accumbens; Shell = shell of nucleus accumbens; Cpu = caudate putamen; SN = substantia nigra; VTA = ventral tegmentum. On each section A indicates the anterior coordinate, measured in millimeters from bregma. (From Tanda et al., 1997.)

that drug. Dopamine release in the nucleus accumbens is triggered by a variety of stimuli that are of significance to the animal—including food and sex. The ability of THC to activate opioid mechanisms also does not mean that THC is equivalent to heroin. Clearly, animals and humans can readily distinguish the distinct subjective experiences elicited by the two drugs, and THC or other cannabinoids do not mimic the severe physical dependence and withdrawal signs associated with chronic heroin use. Nevertheless, there is growing evidence that the naturally occurring opioid and cannabinoid systems represent parallel and sometimes overlapping mechanisms. Rats made dependent on heroin and then challenged with the opiate antagonist naloxone exhibit a strong withdrawal syndrome, with various characteristic behavioral features—for example, "wet dog shakes," teeth chattering, writhing, jumping, and diarrhea. Interestingly, some of these features are seen in a milder form if heroin-dependent animals are challenged with rimonabant. Conversely, rats treated repeatedly with high doses of cannabinoids will exhibit mild signs of withdrawal when challenged with the opiate antagonist naloxone. More support for the concept of a link between the cannabinoid and opioid systems in the brain has come from CB-1 receptor knockout mice (Ledent et al., 1999; reviewed by Valverde et al., 2005). These animals survive quite normally without the CB-1 receptor, but as expected they are unable to show any of the normal CNS responses to THC (analgesia, sedation, and hypothermia). Interestingly, the mice are also less responsive to morphine. Although morphine was still analgesic, it was less likely to be self-administered, and the mice displayed a milder opiate withdrawal syndrome.

Further support for the existence of a genuine cannabis withdrawal syndrome in animals came from De Fonseca et al. (1997), who reported that there were elevated levels of the stress-related chemical corticotropin-releasing factor (CRF) in rat brain when rats were withdrawn from treatment for 2 weeks with the potent cannabinoid HU-210. Elevated levels of brain CRF were also seen in animals during withdrawal from alcohol, cocaine, and heroin. The association of withdrawal with unpleasant anxiety and stress reactions is perhaps one reason why people continue to use drugs of dependence.

Repeated dosing with cannabis clearly leads to dependence and withdrawal in animals, and these phenomena resemble those seen after treatment with other drugs that possess addictive properties. The animal studies, however, tell us little about how serious a problem this may represent for human cannabis users Such information can only come from human studies, some of which will be described in later chapters. (For reviews see Pertwee, 1991; and Lichtman and Martin, 2005.)

# 5

*Medical Uses
of Marijuana—Fact
or Fantasy?*

# Historical

Cannabis has been used as a medicine for thousands of years (Lewin, 1931; Walton, 1938; Robinson, 1996). The Chinese compendium of herbal medicines, the *Pen T'sao Kang Mu*, first published around 2800 B.C., recommended cannabis for the treatment of constipation, gout, malaria, rheumatism, and menstrual problems. Chinese herbal medicine texts continued to recommend cannabis preparations for many centuries. Among other things, its pain-relieving properties were exploited to relieve the pain of surgical operations.

Indian medicine has almost as long a history of using cannabis. The ancient medical text the *Atharva Veda*, which dates from 2000–1400 B.C., mentions *bhang* (the Indian term for marijuana), and further reference is made to this in the writings of Panini (ca. 300 B.C.) (Chopra and Chopra, 1957).

There appears to be no doubt that the cannabis plant was believed by the ancient Aryan settlers of India to possesses sedative, cooling, and febrifuge properties. (Chopra and Chopra, 1957)

In the ancient Ayurvedic system of medicine cannabis played an important role in Hindu materia medica, and continues to be used by Ayurvedic practitioners today. In various medieval Ayurvedic texts cannabis leaves and resin are recommended as a decongestant, an astringent, as soothing, and as capable of stimulating appetite and promoting digestion. Cannabis was also used to induce sleep and as an anaesthetic for surgical operations. It was also considered to have aphrodisiac properties and was recommended for this purpose.

In Arab medicine and in Muslim India frequent mention is also made of *hashish* (cannabis resin) and *benj* (marijuana). They were used to treat gonorrhea, diarrhea, and asthma and as an appetite stimulant and analgesic. In Indian folk medicine bhang and ganja (cannabis resin) were recommended as stimulants to improve staying power under conditions of severe exertion or fatigue. Poultices applied to wounds and sores were believed to promote healing or to act as an anodyne and sedative when applied to areas of inflammation (e.g., piles). Extracts of ganja were used to promote sleep and to treat painful neuralgias, migraine, and menstrual pain. Numerous concoctions containing extracts of cannabis together with various other herbal medicines continue to be used in rural Indian folk medicine today, with a variety of different medical indications including dyspepsia, diarrhea, sprue, dysentery, fever, renal colic, dysmenorrhea, cough, and asthma. Cannabis-based tonics with aphrodisiac claims are also popular. The use of cannabis-based medicines has declined rapidly in India in recent years, however, as more reliable Western-style medicines have become more generally available.

Cannabis or *hemp* was also popular in folk medicine in medieval Europe and was mentioned as a healing plant in herbals such as those by William Turner, Mattioli, and Dioscobas Taberaemontanus (Booth, 2003). One of the most famous herbals, written by Nicholas Culpepper (1616–1654), recommended that:

> …an emulsion of decoction of the seed…eases the colic and always the troublesome humours in the bowels and stays bleeding at the mouth, nose and other places.

It was not until the middle of the nineteenth century, however, that cannabis-based medicines were taken up by mainstream Western medicine. This can be attributed almost entirely to the work of a young Irish doctor, William O'Shaughnessy, serving with the Bengal Medical Service of the East India Company (Booth, 2003). He had observed first hand the many uses of cannabis in Indian medicine, and had himself conducted a series of animal experiments to characterize its effects and establish what doses could be tolerated. His experiments confirmed that cannabis was remarkably safe. Despite many escalations of dose it did not kill any of his experimental animals. O'Shaughnessy felt confident to go on to conduct studies in patients suffering from seizures, rheumatism, tetanus, and rabies. He found what appeared to be clear evidence that cannabis could relieve pain and act as a muscle relaxant and an anticonvulsant. The 30-year-old O'Shaughnessy reported his findings in a remarkable monograph, first published in Calcutta in 1839 and reprinted as a 40-page article in the Transactions of the Medical and Physical Society of Calcutta in 1842

(O'Shaughnessy, 1842). His report rapidly attracted interest from clinicians throughout Europe. As a result of his careful studies, O'Shaughnessy felt able to recommend cannabis, particularly as an "anticonvulsive remedy of the greatest value." He brought back a quantity of cannabis to England in 1842 and Peter Squire on Oxford Street, London, was responsible for converting imported cannabis resin into a medicinal extract and distributing it to a large number of physicians, under O'Shaughnessy's directions.

O'Shaughnessy was a remarkable Victorian genius (Moon, 1967). Before moving to India, he undertook a series of experimental inquiries in Newcastle-upon-Tyne into the composition of the blood in cholera and concluded correctly that there was dehydration and salt loss, and he advocated treatment designed to replace these. O'Shaughnessy never himself put these ideas to the test, but they were rapidly taken up by physicians and found to be effective. Cholera was a common and deadly infectious disease in nineteenth-century cities, which lacked modern sanitation systems. His ideas form the basis of the *fluid replacement therapy*, which, to this day, is the basis of treatment for the catastrophic loss of salts and water from the blood that is a key feature of cholera and other diseases that induce severe diarrhea. On moving to India in 1833, O'Shaughnessy began his studies of cannabis described above, and in 1841 he published an important textbook of chemistry and was made professor of chemistry at the Medical College in Calcutta; 2 years later, at the remarkably young age of 34, he was elected a Fellow of the Royal Society in London. He was subsequently instrumental in constructing thousands of miles of telegraph lines in India, which proved to be of critical importance for communication in this vast part of the British Empire. By the time O'Shaughnessy retired to England in 1860, at the age of 51, there were 11,000 miles of telegraph lines in India and 150 offices in operation. Within 10 years telegraph links to London would be established.

Following O'Shaughnessy's advocacy of cannabis and the availability of the medicinal extract, it became popular for a while in British medical circles. Many doctors began to experiment with cannabis as a new form of treatment, and reports appeared in medical journals describing its application in a variety of conditions, including menstrual cramps, asthma, childbirth, quinsy, cough, insomnia, and migraine headaches, and even in the treatment of withdrawal from opium. Cannabis extract and tincture appeared in the British Pharmacopoeia and were available for more than 100 years:

British Pharmaceutical Codex 1949:
EXTRACTUM CANNABIS
(Ext. Cannab.)
Extract of Cannabis:
Cannabis in coarse powder 1,000 g
Alcohol (90%)....................a sufficient quantity
Exhaust the cannabis by percolation with the alcohol and evaporate to the consistence of a soft extract. Store in well-closed containers, which prevent access of moisture.
Dose: 16 to 60 mg

TINCTURA CANNABIS
(Tinct. Cannab.)
Tincture of Cannabis:
Extract of Cannabis 50 g
Alcohol (90%) to 1,000 ml
Dissolve

Weight per ml at 20°, 0.842 g to 0.852 g
Alcohol content 83 to 87% v/v
Dose 0.3 to 1 ml

In Britain the eminent Victorian physician Sir John Russell Reynolds (Reynolds, 1890) recommended cannabis for sleeplessness, neuralgia, and dysmenorrhea (period pains). It was also experimented with as a means of strengthening uterine contractions in childbirth and in treating opium withdrawal, an increasing problem for Victorian medicine as the uncontrolled consumption of opium created problems of addiction. There was interest in the use of cannabis in the treatment of the insane, following reports by Dr. Jean Jacques Moreau in Paris of this possibility. But there was also concern that excessive use of cannabis could lead to insanity, a concern that persisted for many years—leading, among other things, to the Indian Hemp Drugs Commission's review of the use of cannabis in India at the end of the nineteenth century (see Chapter 8), and revived again recently with claims that the teenage use of cannabis may lead to subsequent mental illness (see Chapter 6).

Although Dr. Reynolds is said to have prescribed cannabis to Queen Victoria to treat her period pains, cannabis never really became popular in British medicine and was used only infrequently. Difficulties in obtaining supplies and the inconsistent results obtained with different preparations of the drug made it hard to use. Because of the lack of any quality control to allow the preparation of standardized batches of the medicine, patients were likely to receive a dose that either had no effect or caused unwanted intoxication. Cannabis was never as reliable and widely used as opium — the mainstay of the Victorian medicine cabinet. Cannabis fell so far out of favor that it was the lack of any continuing medical use as much as any other factor that led to its removal from the *British Pharmacopoeia* by the middle of the twentieth century.

In America, cannabis was already known even before O'Shaughnessy made it popular in Europe. It was first introduced into homeopathic medicine, as described in the *New Homeopathic Pharmacopoeia and Posology or the Preparation of Homeopathic Medicines* (Jahr, 1842). Cannabis came to the notice of psychiatrists also, who experimented with its use in treating the mentally ill. By 1854 the U.S. Dispensatory began to list cannabis among the nation's medicinals, and gave the following remarkably accurate description of its properties:

> Medical Properties: Extract of hemp is a powerful narcotic, causing exhilaration, intoxication, delirious hallucinations, and, in its subsequent action drowsiness and stupor, with little effect upon the circulation. It is asserted also to act as a decided aphrodisiac, to increase the appetite, and occasionally to induce the cataleptic state. In morbid states of the system, it has been found to produce sleep, to allay spasm, to compose nervous inquietude, and to relieve pain. In these respects it resembles opium in its operation; but it differs from that narcotic in not diminishing the appetite, checking the secretions, or constipating the bowels. It is much less certain in its effects; but may sometimes be preferably employed, when opium is contraindicated by its nauseating or constipating effects, or its disposition to cause headache, and to check the bronchial secretion. The complaints to which it has been

specially recommended are neuralgia, gout, tetanus, hydrophobia, epidemic cholera, convulsions, chorea, hysteria, mental depression, insanity, and uterine hemorrhage. Dr Alexander Christison, of Edinburgh, has found it to have the property of hastening and increasing the contractions of the uterus in delivery, and has employed it with advantage for this purpose. It acts very quickly, and without anesthetic effect. It appears, however, to exert this influence only in a certain proportion of cases. (Wood and Bache, 1854)

Although cannabis continued to attract the interest of psychiatrists, it did not become widely popular with American doctors. During the Civil War it was used to treat diarrhea and dysentery among the soldiers, but as a medicine cannabis had too many shortcomings. As British doctors had found, the potency of commercial preparations varied from pharmacist to pharmacist as there was no means of standardizing the preparations for their content of the active drug. In addition, the drug was not water soluble and so, unlike morphine, cannabis could not be given by injection. The hypodermic syringe was invented in the late nineteenth century and was immediately popular with doctors and patients for administering instant remedies. There is a certain mystique associated with the ritual of an injection—even today many Japanese patients prefer their medicines to be administered in this way. Cannabis had to be given by mouth and took some time to take effect. The doctor might have to remain with his patient for more than an hour after giving the drug, in order to make sure not only that it was having the desired effect, but also that the dosage had not been too high.

A succinct and perceptive summary of the rise and fall of cannabis in nineteenth-century medicine is given by Walton (1938, p. 152):

The popularity of the hemp drugs can be attributed partly to the fact that they were introduced before the synthetic hypnotics and analgesics. Chloral hydrate was not introduced until 1869 and was followed in the next 30 years by paraldehyde, sulfonal and the barbitals. Antipyrine and acetanilide, the first of their particular group of analgesics [aspirin-like drugs], were introduced about 1884 [aspirin, not until 1899]. For general sedative and analgesic purposes, the only drugs commonly used at this time were the morphine derivatives and their disadvantages were very well known. In fact, the most attractive feature of the hemp narcotics was probably the fact that they did not exhibit

certain of the notorious disadvantages of the opiates. The hemp narcotics do
not constipate at all, they more often increase rather than decrease appetite,
they do not particularly depress the respiratory center even in large doses, they
rarely or never cause pruritis or cutaneous eruption and, most importantly,
the liability of developing addiction is very much less than with the opiates.
These features were responsible for the rapid rise in popularity of the
drug. Several features can be recognised as contributing to the gradual decline of popularity. Cannabis does not usually produce analgesia or relax
spastic conditions without producing cortical effects and, in fact, these cortical effects usually predominate. The actual degree of analgesia produced is
much less than with the opiates. Most important, the effects are irregular due
to marked variations in individual susceptibility and probably also to variable
absorption of the gummy resin.

Pharmaceutical companies, nevertheless, tried to make use of cannabis as a medicine and it was included in dozens of proprietary medicines,
which were available over the counter in the nineteenth century and the
early years of this century. These included the stomach remedy Chloro-
dyne (which also contained morphine) (Squibb Co.), Corn Collodium
(Squibb Co.), Dr. Brown's Sedative Tablets, and One Day Cough Cure
(Eli Lilly Co). The company Grimault and Sons marketed cannabis cigarettes as a remedy for asthma. By 1937, when cannabis was removed from
medical use in the United States, some 28 different medicines contained it
as an ingredient—many of them with no indication of its presence.

## The Modern Revival of Interest in
## Cannabis-Based Medicines

During most of the twentieth century there was little interest in the use of
cannabis in Western medicine, and such use has been legally prohibited
since 1937 in the United States and since the 1970s in Britain and most of
Europe. In all of these countries cannabis was classified as a Schedule 1
drug (i.e., a dangerous addictive narcotic with no recognized medical uses).
As cannabis became an increasingly popular recreational drug during the
1960s and 1970s, however, more and more people were exposed to it, and

during the 1980s and 1990s there was an increasing interest in medical applications. Many normally law-abiding citizens in the developed world started to use cannabis illegally for therapy. The groups most commonly involved in such illegal self-medication were those suffering from chronic pain conditions unresponsive to other pain-relieving drugs. A recent survey of more than 2,000 self-selected users of medicinal cannabis in the United Kingdom showed that multiple sclerosis (MS), neuropathy and other chronic pain states, arthritis, and depression were the most common indications (Ware et al., 2005), and similar results were obtained in a survey of the medical use of cannabis in the Netherlands, where it is legal (Gorter et al., 2005). Data from British Multiple Sclerosis Society questionnaires suggested that 30% of patients had tried cannabis and 10% reported regular use (Royal College of Physicians, 2005). Most of the patients who take cannabis for medical reasons smoke marijuana—in contrast to the earlier use of the drug in Western medicine, which was invariably taken by mouth and not smoked.

With many centuries of experience of cannabis as a safe medicine, and with thousands of patients in Western countries convinced of the benefits of the drug, why is there any problem? Why do Western governments not agree to make it legally available for doctors to prescribe for their patients? Governments have clearly stated political reasons for withholding such consent, as they do not wish to "give the wrong message" to young people. If teenagers see governments approving cannabis as a drug that is safe to use medically, would this not encourage even greater illicit recreational use? Some critics see the campaign for medical marijuana as part of an overall campaign by some groups to legalize cannabis. As drug czar Barry McCaffrey put it in a press release on November 15, 1996:

> There could be no worse message to young people.... Just when the nation is trying its hardest to educate teenagers not to use psychoactive drugs, now they are being told that marijuana is a medicine.

But the Institute of Medicine (1999) report put the opposing view:

> There is a broad social concern that sanctioning the medical use of marijuana might increase its use among the general population. At this point

there are no convincing data to support this concern. The existing data are consistent with the idea that this would not be a problem if the medical use of marijuana were as closely regulated as other medications with abuse potential.

But are there any scientific reasons to withhold a safe and effective medicine from patients? The evidence for and against medicinal cannabis has been the subject of a number of expert reviews during the past decade. A report by the British Medical Association on the Therapeutic Uses of Cannabis published in 1997 was followed by the UK House of Lords enquiry into cannabis (1998), the U.S. Institute of Medicine's *Marijuana and Medicine* (1999), and most recently the British Royal College of Physicians' *Cannabis and Cannabis-based Medicines* (2005).

The problem is that although cannabis has been used in human medicine for some 4,000 years, we have not until very recently had rigorous scientific evidence for either its safety or its effectiveness except in a few isolated instances. The fact of the matter is that many folk medicines and herbal remedies have no real beneficial medical effects; they are used because of tradition and folklore, and in many cases if patients show some improvement in their symptoms this says more for the power of suggestion than the efficacy of the medicines. This is seen par excellence with homeopathic medicines. These consist of a variety of natural ingredients used in very dilute form. Homeopathic medicine has no scientific rationale. Nevertheless, if patients believe that a treatment will benefit them, this belief and the optimism with which it imbues them can have powerful effects on the course of an illness.

The effects of homeopathic and herbal medicines and various other alternative medicine approaches most likely involve the well-documented placebo effect. If people are given a tablet or capsule that is identical to that containing a genuine medicine but that contains no active ingredients other than sugar or some other inert powder, they will often report that they feel better. This even extends to the treatment of severe pain, where patients receiving placebo may report pain relief. Some years ago Jon Levine and Howard Fields, researchers at the University of California in San Francisco, conducted some ingenious experiments that shed some light on the mysterious placebo effect. They studied groups of students who had attended the student dental clinic for the surgical removal of wisdom teeth. The students were told that they would receive either an inactive placebo or the powerful painkiller morphine. Two hours after recovering from the anaesthetic, the subjects who had volunteered to take part in this study received an intravenous injection of either morphine or a saline placebo. To ensure that the investigator did not inadvertently reveal whether the subjects were receiving morphine or placebo, the study was blinded—that is, neither the subjects nor the physician knew which subjects were receiving the active drug. This information was coded and held by someone not involved directly in the experiment and the code was only broken when the experiment was complete. After a dental operation most people experience pain that increases gradually over a period of several hours. The subjects who received morphine reported that their pain was either stable or decreased. Those who received the placebo saline injection, however, fell into two groups. About two thirds of them showed no response and their pain increased gradually over the course of the study, but about one third of the placebo group was classified as "responders" since they reported pain relief that was equivalent to subjects who had received a moderate dose of morphine (Levine et al., 1979) (Fig. 5.1). In a subsequent study it was found that the drug naloxone, which acts as a potent antagonist of the actions of morphine at opiate receptors, could prevent the placebo response in placebo responders, but it had no effect in placebo nonresponders. How could naloxone block the effect of a drug that the placebo group had not received? The answer seems to be that the mere expectation of pain relief from an injection that might contain morphine was by itself sufficient in some people to activate the body's own natural opiate system, causing the release of the morphine-like chemicals known as endorphins in the brain and spinal cord. This produced pain relief, but the endorphins were ineffective in the presence of naloxone, which blocks the receptors through which they act.

The San Francisco study gives us some hint of how some genuine placebo effects may be explained. It also illustrates some of the principles underlying modern clinical trials. The introduction of new medicines for human use requires that they fulfill internationally agreed-upon criteria

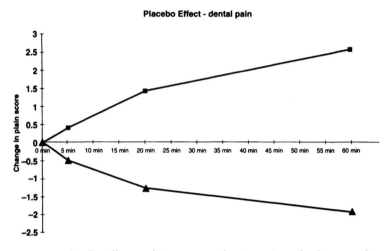

**Figure 5.1.** Placebo effect. Subjects received an injection of either morphine or saline (placebo) in a blinded manner 2 hours after dental surgery, and were asked to rate their pain scores on an arbitrary scale for the subsequent hour. Data are shown only for the group receiving placebo. Of 107 patients in this group, 42 (39%) were rated as placebo responders. Whereas nonresponders experienced an increasing level of pain (filled squares), the placebo responders either reported some degree of pain relief (filled triangles) or their pain remained unchanged (data not shown). (Redrawn from Levine et al., 1979.)

for safety and effectiveness laid down by the various government regulatory agencies responsible for the approval of new medicines. The effectiveness of the medicine in treating a particular illness has to be established in controlled clinical trials. *Controlled* means comparing the test drug with an inactive placebo prepared in such a manner that it cannot be distinguished from the active medicine. In a double-blind, randomized, placebo-controlled trial neither the patient nor the doctor or nurse knows whether active drug or placebo is given to any particular patient. Patients are randomly allocated to placebo and test drug groups to avoid any possible bias in the selection of those who are to receive the active drug. This information is held in coded form by a person not actively involved in the conduct of the trial and is not made available until the trial has ended. The outcome of the trial should involve objective measurements wherever possible, using predetermined outcome measures or endpoints. The success or failure of the trial is measured by criteria established in a written trial protocol before the start of the trial. Because individual patients will inevitably vary in their response to drug or placebo, the trial should include a sufficiently large number of subjects to provide statistically significant differences in outcome measures between the placebo and drug-treated groups. It is not uncommon for a clinical trial to involve hundreds or even thousands of subjects.

There are a number of variants on clinical trial design. For example, it is not always necessary to use separate groups of patients to assess test-drug or placebo responses. In the so-called *crossover* trial design the same patients receive placebo and test drug at different stages during the trial and are crossed over from one to the other after a wash-out period (to ensure removal of any active drug from the body). The test drug or placebo is given to different patients in random order, so that the trial remains double blind.

These principles of clinical trial design, although they may appear to be simply common sense, are relatively new. It is only in the past 50 years that the concept of the controlled clinical trial has become generally accepted. It can be applied not only to the testing of new medicines, but also to the effectiveness of any new medical procedure.

The reasons for insisting on these elaborate scientifically controlled trials was the growing realization that the expectations of both doctor and patient can influence the outcome of a clinical trial, even though neither may be consciously aware of this. The importance of the placebo effect means that this has to be built into the design of clinical trials. Not all human illnesses will show the same degree of susceptibility to the placebo effect; such treatment is most likely to affect the outcome of conditions in which there are strong psychological or psychosomatic components and less likely to influence the outcome of infectious diseases or cancer. Placebo effects are particularly prominent in the treatment of such psychiatric conditions as anxiety and depression, and are often seen in illnesses in which the patient has failed to gain any benefit from existing conventional medicines. Such patients are often desperately seeking new treatments, which they want to work.

There is a real possibility that some of the medical benefits claimed by patients who are self-medicating with cannabis could lie in that category. The patients are usually those for whom conventional medicine has failed and they are turning to alternative medicine for relief from their symptoms. Cannabis has the added attraction to many of being a natural and herbal remedy, embedded in centuries of folklore and folk medicine. At the moment very few of the medical indications for which herbal cannabis is illegally used can be substantiated by data from scientifically controlled clinical trials. The thousands of patients who are currently self-medicating rely almost entirely on word-of-mouth anecdotal evidence and their own personal experiences of the drug. Anecdotal evidence, however, is not reliable and cannot be used to persuade regulatory agencies to approve cannabis as a medicine. To the nonscientist this is hard to understand. The often moving personal accounts of individuals who report the benefits they have derived from herbal cannabis are so compelling—what more is needed? Professor Grinspoon at Harvard has long been a passionate advocate of cannabis-based medicines, and has given a fascinating series of accounts of patients' individual experiences (Grinspoon and Bakalar, 1993).

Fortunately, the past decade has seen a new era of controlled trials of cannabis-based medicines, yielding enough positive evidence to persuade government regulatory agencies in some advanced countries (Canada and Spain) to give formal approval for the use of these products.

## The Synthetic Cannabinoids

In the sound and fury of the debate about the medical use of herbal cannabis, with strongly held positions on both sides of the argument, it is often forgotten that two cannabis-based medicines are already available by prescription to patients on both sides of the Atlantic. These are the synthetic cannabinoids dronabinol (trade name Marinol) and nabilone (trade name Cesamet). Although they have not proved very popular, the medical use of these compounds, unlike herbal cannabis, is backed up by a substantial body of scientific evidence from clinical trials, and the compounds have satisfied the strict requirements of the U.S. Food and Drug Administration (FDA) and the corresponding European agencies for approval as human medicines.

## Dronabinol (Marinol)

Dronabinol is the generic name given to synthetic delta-9-tetrahydrocannabinol (THC) (see Fig. 2.1). It is marketed as the medical product known as Marinol. Drugs are given an *official generic name*—which is used when describing the compound in the scientific literature—and the company that markets the drug usually gives it a separate *trade name*. The same drug may be marketed by more than one company under different trade names, but each compound can only possess one generic name.

One of the problems in using dronabinol as a medicine is that the pure compound is a viscous pale-yellow resin, which is almost completely insoluble in water. This makes it impossible to prepare as a simple tablet and it cannot be dissolved for administration as an intravenous injection. Marinol is, therefore, prepared by dissolving dronabinol in a small quantity of harmless sesame oil in a soft gelatin capsule (containing 2.5, 5, or 10 mg dronabinol). These capsules are easily swallowed and absorption is almost complete (90% to 95%), but because much of the active drug is metabolized during passage of the blood from the gut via the liver, only 10% to 20% of the administered dose reaches the general circulation. Effects begin after 30 minutes to 1 hour and reach a peak at 2 to 4 hours, with duration of action of 4 to 6 hours, although the appetite-stimulating effects of the drug may persist for up to 24 hours. Considerable quantities of the psychoactive metabolite 11-hydroxy-THC (see Chapter 2) are formed in the liver, and this metabolite is present in blood at approximately the same level as the parent drug, with a similar duration of action.

Two medical indications have been approved for dronabinol. The first of these is its use to counteract the nausea and vomiting frequently associated with cancer chemotherapy; the other is as an appetite stimulant to counteract the AIDS wasting syndrome, as described below (for review see Plasse et al., 1991). The annual sales of Marinol in the United States were $78 million in 2004. About 80% of prescriptions are for HIV/AIDS patients, 10% for cancer chemotherapy, and 10% for a range of other purposes. The possibility that medical supplies of dronabinol might be diverted to illicit use has been a concern, but there is very little evidence that this has happened. Dronabinol has little value as a street drug. The onset of action is slow and gradual and its effects are unappealing to regular marijuana smokers; it has a very low abuse potential. Because of the low dependence liability, the U.S. Drug Enforcement Agency reclassified Marinol to the less restrictive Schedule III in 1998, although pure THC remains a Schedule 1 substance.

## Nabilone (Cesamet)

During the 1970s a number of pharmaceutical companies carried out research on synthetic analogs of THC to see whether it might be possible to dissociate the desired medical effects from the psychotropic actions. On the whole this quest proved disappointing (see Chapter 2), and in retrospect this may have been inevitable since we now believe that both the desired effects and the intoxicant actions of THC result from activation of the same CB-1 receptors in the central nervous system. Only one company persisted with this research long enough to produce a marketed product—nabilone (Cesamet), (see Fig. 2.2). Nabilone is a potent analog of THC, which scientists at the Eli Lilly Company believed might have an improved separation of the desired therapeutic effects from psychotropic actions. Unlike dronabinol, nabilone is a stable crystalline solid, and for human use the drug is prepared in solid form in capsules containing 1 mg of nabilone that are taken by mouth, and the dose is usually 1 or 2 mg twice a day.

Preliminary clinical studies in the treatment of anxiety gave promising results, but the company decided to focus on the treatment of nausea and vomiting in patients undergoing cancer chemotherapy as the primary target. They carried out the most complete series of controlled clinical trials so far undertaken on any cannabinoid, as described below (for review see Lemberger, 1985).

## Medical Targets for Cannabis

Many medical uses have been claimed for cannabis, but in most cases scientific evidence for efficacy is lacking, or new and easier-to-use medicines have become available. The following sections are arranged in order of priority—the highest being given where the best evidence is available and alternative medicines are few. (For reviews see British Medical Association [1997]; Institute of Medicine [1999]; Royal College of Physicians [2005]; and Robson [2005].)

### Multiple Sclerosis

MS is the most common disabling nervous system disease of young adults, with an estimated 85,000 living with the condition in the United Kingdom and more than 250,000 in the United States. MS is a progressive, degenerative disease in which the brain and the spinal cord nerves are damaged by the gradual destruction of myelin, the protective, insulating layer of fatty tissue that normally coats nerve fibres. The precise cause of the disease is not known, but it is thought to represent an autoimmune condition, in which the body's immune system becomes inappropriately sensitized to some component of myelin—leading to its attack and progressive damage by the immune system. The disease usually progresses in stages, with periods of remission between, but it is ultimately life threatening. The symptoms are very variable, depending on which particular nerves or regions of the central nervous system (CNS) are damaged, but it often manifests itself with symptoms of muscle spasticity, pain, and bladder and bowel dysfunction. The British Multiple Sclerosis Society reported the results of a survey of their 35,000 members to the House of Lords Science and Technology Committee Cannabis Report in 1998. Fatigue was the most frequent symptom reported by 95% of patients, followed by balance problems (84%), muscle weakness (81%), incontinence (76%), muscle spasms (66%), pain (61%), and tremor (35%).

The treatment of MS has improved radically in recent years with the introduction of new medicines that slow the rate of progression of the disease, β-interferon and the antibody natalizumab, but neither of these represents a complete cure (http://www.mult-sclerosis.org). There are also several medicines available to treat the symptoms of MS, but none is wholly effective. The drugs baclofen and diazepam (Valium) help to relax muscle spasms by activating receptors for the inhibitory chemical messenger γ-aminobutyric acid (GABA) in the brain and spinal cord, thus counteracting overactivity in the flow of excitatory signals to muscles. Both drugs may cause side effects, including sedation, drowsiness, and confusion. Dantrolene acts directly on muscle to dampen the force of contraction but can cause serious side effects (headache, drowsiness, dizziness, malaise, and nausea). Oxybutynin, flavoxate, and propantheline can be helpful in controlling urinary incontinence; they block the actions of the chemical signal acetylcholine that triggers bladder emptying. All of these drugs may cause dry mouth, blurred vision, constipation, and difficulty in initiating urine flow as side effects. Chronic pain in MS sufferers is often hard to treat, but drugs used in the treatment of epilepsy (carbamazepine, phenytoin) or depression (amitriptyline) and even opiates are sometimes used. Despite the relatively large numbers of patients with MS, it has not attracted much attention from pharmaceutical research companies. The muscle relaxant tizanidine launched in the United Kingdom in late 1997 was the first new drug to receive approval for the treatment of muscle spasticity in 20 years.

MS represents a promising target for cannabis-based medicines (Consroe and Snider, 1986). Anecdotal reports suggest that cannabis can relieve not only the muscle spasms and the pain they cause, but in some patients it can also improve bladder control. The sedative properties of cannabis may also offer sound sleep to patients whose sleep is otherwise frequently disturbed by painful muscle spasms and the frequent need to urinate. The use of cannabis in the treatment of various types of painful muscle spasms has a sound scientific rationale. CB-1 receptors are found in particularly high density in those regions of the brain that are involved in the control of muscle function—the basal ganglia and the cerebellum. The receptors are densely located on output neurons in the outflow relay stations of the basal ganglia (substantia nigra and globus pallidus), where they are well placed to affect the control of movements. Activation of the cannabinoid receptors is known to suppress movements and can lead to a condition of catalepsy, in which the person or animal may remain conscious but immobile for considerable periods. It is not surprising, therefore, that cannabinoid drugs possess antispastic properties. In an animal model of MS in mice (allergic encephalomyelitis), the animal's immune system is sensitized to a component of its own myelin and there is progressive nervous system damage accompanied by muscle tremor. This and other symptoms in this animal model can be suppressed by treatment with THC (Baker et al., 2001; Arevola-Martin et al., 2003). In this model repeated treatment with THC also has the effect of slowing down the development of the syndrome—suggesting that cannabinoids might even be able to alter the course of an autoimmune disease, perhaps because of their ability to dampen immune system activity.

Until recently there were only eight published clinical trials of cannabis in MS, involving a total of less than 100 subjects worldwide, and the results were equivocal (for review see Pryce and Baker, 2005). Most of the evidence supporting the use of cannabis in MS was anecdotal. But there have been more systematic surveys of MS patients in the United Kingdom, Germany, Canada, and the Netherlands who admitted to self-medicating with smoked marijuana (Atha, 2005). A majority of the respondents reported that marijuana improved their spasticity, muscle pain, nighttime spasticity, leg pain at night, depression, and tremor. Many also reported improvements in anxiety, daytime spasticity, tingling, numbness, facial pain, muscle weakness, and weight loss.

The past few years, however, have seen the first large-scale controlled trials of cannabis in MS. The largest of these, the CAMS study (Cannabis in Multiple Sclerosis), was sponsored by the British Medical Research Council (Zajicek et al., 2003). The double-blind placebo-controlled trial involved more than 600 MS patients, randomly allocated to three treatment groups, all of whom received oral capsules containing placebo, pure THC (2.5 mg), or a standardized herbal cannabis extract (2.5 mg THC + 1.25 mg cannabidiol). An initial period of dose finding adjusted the dose to avoid CNS side effects (range 3 to 10 capsules per day), and treatment then continued daily for 15 weeks. The primary outcome measure was an objective assessment of limb spasticity, undertaken by a doctor manipulating a lower limb and assessing the degree of muscle spasticity on a 4-point scale—the Ashworth scale. All patients initially had Ashworth scores of 2 or above, and in the first 15-week phase of the study there was no significant reduction in these scores in response to THC or cannabis extract (Fig. 5.2). The choice of the Ashworth scale as the primary outcome measure, however, has since been questioned (Pryce and Baker, 2005). It has yielded negative results even with trials of accepted treatments for MS spasticity (baclofen and tizanidine). Despite the lack of objective evidence for an effect on spasticity, the subjective assessments reported by the patients treated with cannabis or THC showed statistically significant improvements in spasticity, muscle spasms, improved sleep, and reductions in pain, and there was objective evidence for improved mobility in a timed walk test. More encouraging were the data from the follow-up phase of the CAMS study, in which two thirds of the original patients opted to continue in the trial for up to 1 year. At this stage there was a significant improvement in the Ashworth spasticity scores and in measures of overall disability (Zajicek et al., 2005), although only the group treated with pure THC and not those treated with herbal

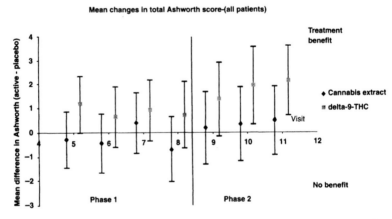

Figure 5.2. Changes in Ashworth scores (measure of limb spasticity) in first and second phases of CAMS clinical trial of cannabis extract or THC in multiple sclerosis. Data show changes in Ashworth scale from placebo in treated groups. Only the THC data from THC-treated patients in Phase 2 were statistically significant. (Redrafted from Zajicek et al., 2005; kindly supplied by Dr. J.P. Zajicek.)

cannabis extract showed significant improvement in the Ashworth scores. This might suggest that other components in the complex mixture of substances present in the plant extract were actually tending to negate the beneficial effects of THC. Further analysis of the CAMS follow-up data suggest that cannabis may have beneficial effects beyond symptom relief in MS. The reason that beneficial effects on spasticity were not seen until treatment was continued for 1 year may be because the cannabinoid had slowed the progression of the disease—as had been suggested previously on the basis of animal experiments (Baker et al., 2001; Arevola-Martin et al., 2003). This hypothesis is currently being tested in further clinical trials, which may extend for up to 5 years of treatment. The CAMS study remains the largest controlled clinical trial of cannabis ever undertaken.

In addition to MS, marijuana is also used illegally by other groups of patients who suffer from disabling illnesses that are accompanied by painful muscle spasms. These include cerebral palsy, torticollis, various dystonias, and spinal injury. Survey data from patients suffering from spinal injuries indicated that more than 90% reported marijuana helped improve symptoms of muscle spasms of the arms or legs and improved urinary control and function.

The official approval of the first cannabis-based medicine to undergo conventional clinical development and to be approved as a prescription medicine for treating MS has relied on the commercial development of such a product by the British pharmaceutical company GW Pharmaceuticals (http://www.gwpharm.com). Sativex is a standardized extract from cloned cannabis plants grown under controlled conditions indoors. One strain of plants produces principally THC (>90% of total cannabinoids) while another yields mainly cannabidiol (>85%). Extracts from the two strains are blended to produce Sativex, containing a 50/50 mixture of THC and cannabidiol. Sativex is delivered by a metered spray device under the tongue or onto the cheek inside the mouth. This avoids smoking or the unreliable oral route and leads to a relatively efficient absorption into the abundant blood vessels in the oral cavity, although it still takes 3 to 4 hours for peak plasma levels of THC to be attained. Patients adjust their individual dose to avoid unwanted side effects; this usually results in the administration of 8 to 12 sprays per day, each delivering 2.7 mg

THC and 2.5 mg cannabidiol, giving an average daily dose of 22 to 32 mg THC (Robson, 2005). More than 700 MS patients have been involved in controlled trials of Sativex (Robson, 2005; Barnes, 2006). The results of one small, 4-week trial involving 66 MS patients showed significant improvements in self-rated pain scores and reduced sleep disturbance in the treated versus placebo groups (Rog et al., 2005). Although the changes in pain scores were small, they were highly valued by the patients, who reported overall benefits from the treatment. These results were sufficient for Sativex to gain approval in Canada in 2005 as a prescription medicine for the treatment of neuropathic pain in MS—a milestone event. Other trials have confirmed the efficacy of Sativex in treating the symptoms of pain, sleep disturbance, and spasticity. An analysis of the data from two trials that focused on spasticity as the primary outcome measure showed significant benefits, with 42% of patients on Sativex reporting at least a 30% improvement compared with 28% in the placebo group (Wade et al., 2005). A small open-label (unblinded) trial of Sativex in MS patients showed it to be effective in improving bladder control both at night and during the day (Brady et al., 2004). A follow-up analysis of patient diaries from the CAMS study also found a significant reduction in incontinence episodes in patients receiving the active treatment (Freeman et al., 2006). Thus, Sativex appears to have significant benefits in treating some of the most common symptoms of MS, confirming earlier anecdotal reports. In the various short-term trials Sativex was safe and well tolerated. The most common side effects were dizziness, nausea, and fatigue, with surprisingly few reports of unwanted intoxicant effects. A long-term open-label follow-up study with Sativex involved 137 MS patients treated for up to 814 days (average 434 days) (Wade et al., 2006). A total of 58 patients withdrew owing to lack of efficacy or unwanted side effects. In the long-term studies the most common adverse side effects were oral pain, dizziness, diarrhea, and nausea. The oral pain was presumably related to repeat oral dosing with the solvent-containing Sativex spray. For those patients who reported an initial benefit and remained in the trial, the positive effects remained stable over time. The long-term study also showed that there was no tendency for patients to increase the daily dose of Sativex over a period of

82 weeks; nor was there any obvious "withdrawal" syndrome when Sativex treatment was suddenly stopped in 25 patients.

The results with Sativex are clearly an important advance in the modern clinical development of a cannabis-based medicine. However, there are a number of factors that suggest that caution is needed in interpreting the findings. By modern standards the clinical trials with Sativex to date have involved relatively small numbers of patients, although by continuing to amass data from a number of such trials a significant database is being built. A question has also been raised as to whether the clinical trials were adequately blinded. It is difficult to conceal the identity of the active cannabis treatment from patients. Cannabis has obvious psychic effects, which may become apparent to patients in their initial dose-ranging administration of the drug. Even in the CAMS trial 77% of the MS patients receiving active drug accurately guessed that they were receiving this, versus only 50% in the placebo group (Zajicek et al., 2003). Herbal cannabis also has a characteristic smell, which may be recognized easily, particularly by those patients with previous experience of cannabis, even though Sativex contains peppermint oil, which may help to hide the identity of the active drug. However, there were no differences in outcome or reported adverse effects between cannabis-experienced versus cannabis-inexperienced subjects, and an independent statistical review of the Sativex data concluded that there had not been any unblinding.

Pain

As reviewed in Chapter 2, there is an increasing body of evidence from experiments in animals that activation of the cannabinoid system in the central nervous system among other things reduces the sensitivity to pain. Clinical pain comes in many varieties from the severe but usually short-lived pain that follows injury or surgical operation to the chronic and often disabling pain that often accompanies such illnesses as rheumatism, arthritis, and cancer.

Many different analgesic (pain-relieving) medicines are available, from aspirin and the many aspirin-like anti-inflammatory drugs, which act on peripheral inflamed tissues, to morphine, codeine, and other opiates, which act directly on the CNS. None of them is completely satisfactory.

Use of aspirin-like drugs carries with it the danger of irritation and ulceration of the stomach, which can lead to dangerous internal bleeding. Several thousand people die each year because of these side effects. Morphine and other opiates often cause severe constipation and at high doses they can depress respiration and cause death. The repeated use of opiates can lead to the development of tolerance, so that patients become less and less sensitive to the drugs and require increasing doses; some may become dependent on the opiate. As with cannabis, the psychotropic effects of opiates are disturbing rather than pleasurable to most patients. Nowadays many patients are provided with medical devices that permit the self-administration of morphine to counteract chronic pain; they learn to adjust the dose of drug to obtain the maximum pain relief without becoming stuporous and intoxicated.

Some of the most distressing forms of clinical pain are those which arise from damage to nerves or to the spinal cord or brain. This can arise from many different causes, as a consequence of accidental or surgical injury to nerves; in patients with diabetes or AIDS, which often leads to damage in peripheral nerves; in multiple sclerosis as described above; as a result of treatment with powerful cancer chemotherapy drugs that can damage nerves; and in some forms of cancer where the tumor presses on or damages nerve fibers. These so-called *neuropathic* pain syndromes are often long lasting and severe—and they are very hard to treat, as even the most powerful analgesic drugs, the opiates, are generally ineffective. In some cases patients respond to treatment with antiepilepsy drugs such as carbamazepine, phenytoin, or gabapentin or to drugs used more commonly in the treatment of depression such as amitriptyline, but for many sufferers neuropathic pain remains untreatable.

An encouraging feature of the results on animal models is that THC has been reported to be effective as an analgesic in models of neuropathic pain, for example, in rats in which the sciatic nerve (which innervates the hind limb) is damaged surgically, and the partially denervated limb becomes sensitized to pain. Morphine and related opiates have previously been shown to be ineffective in this and other animal models of neuropathic pain.

The historical literature on the medical uses of cannabis has also long stressed its value in the treatment of a variety of painful conditions, but until recently there have been few controlled scientific studies. A number of small clinical trials of orally administered THC have reported mixed results. Campbell et al. (2001) reviewed such studies and concluded:

> Cannabinoids are no more effective than codeine in controlling pain and have depressant effects on the central nervous system that limit their use. Their widespread introduction into clinical practice for pain management is therefore undesirable.... Before cannabinoids can be considered for treating spasticity and neuropathic pain, further valid randomised controlled studies are needed.

Data from such studies have recently become available. There is no test that provides an objective measure of pain. Clinical trials must, therefore, always rely on the patient's own reports. Commonly used subjective measures include numerical (Fig. 5.3) and visual analog scales, often with an 11-point scale from "no pain" to "worst possible pain," which yield daily pain scores for each patient.

Serpell et al. (2005) and Nurmikko et al. (2007) reported results with Sativex in a 4-week randomized, placebo-controlled trial in 125 patients with neuropathic pain accompanied by allodynia. This is a condition in which previously innocuous light stimuli become exquisitely painful. The results showed a significant improvement in pain scores, allodynia, and sleep disturbance in the Sativex-treated group versus the placebo group. In a long-term follow-up study 89 of these patients opted to receive Sativex in an open-label manner. The mean treatment duration was 288 days, but some patients remained on Sativex for more than 2 years. In those patients who remained in the study, pain control and improved sleep was maintained

Select the number that best describes your pain during the past 24 hours.

Circle one number only.

| 0 | 1 | 2 | 3 | 4 | 5 | 6 | 7 | 8 | 9 | 10 |

No Pain                                                           Worst Possible Pain

Figure 5.3. A numerical scale for rating pain.

throughout, although some two thirds of the patients withdrew because of adverse effects or lack of efficacy (Serpell et al., 2006).

In another randomized controlled trial Sativex was tested in a cross-over design (2 weeks on drug, 2 weeks on placebo) in 48 patients suffering from pain due to damage to the nerves innervating the arm and shoulder (Berman et al., 2004). In accidents these nerves can be partly torn from their roots in the spinal cord, leading to a constant crushing and burning pain felt in the affected arm. It is not uncommon for this to persist for many years, making at a difficult condition to treat. There were statistically significant improvements in pain scores and sleep disturbance was reduced. Although the effect of Sativex on pain scores was small (a <1 point improvement on an 11-point self-rated scale), 80% of the patients opted to continue on the cannabis drug in an extension study.

Two larger clinical trials have been completed with Sativex in the treatment of neuropathic pain (GW Pharmaceutical Press Release, January 15, 2007). One involved 246 patients with neuropathic pain accompanied by allodynia, and Sativex again proved significantly better than placebo in reducing pain scores; there were also significant improvements in sleep quality and in the patients' own impression of global change. A second study involved 297 patients with neuropathic pain caused by damage to peripheral nerves in diabetes (a not uncommon complication of the illness). Although Sativex led to an average 30% reduction in pain scores (with one third reporting more than a 50% reduction), the results were not statistically significant because of a large and variable placebo response.

Preliminary results suggest that Sativex may also be effective in treating other types of pain. In a randomized controlled trial in 58 patients with pain caused by rheumatoid arthritis, by comparison with placebo Sativex produced significant improvements in pain and quality of sleep. In addition, there were significant improvements in measures of disease activity — suggesting that there might be a beneficial effect in slowing the disease process as well as in relieving the acute symptoms (Blake et al., 2006).

In another randomized controlled study Sativex proved effective in relieving cancer-related pain in 177 patients with advanced cancer (Johnson et al., 2005), and Sativex was approved in August 2007 by Health Canada for use in the treatment of cancer pain.

These studies have provided scientific evidence to support the historical claims for the effectiveness of cannabis in pain relief. Although the effects of cannabis have usually proved small in magnitude, patients often report them as clinically meaningful. There is as yet no officially approved cannabis-based medicine for the treatment of pain, other than in Canada, where Sativex is approved for the treatment of pain associated with MS and cancer, but such approval is likely to occur eventually in response to an ever-increasing body of positive controlled trial data.

The available data suggest that cannabis-based medicines can benefit patients with certain hard-to-treat pain conditions, although their efficacy is variable and somewhat limited (perhaps comparable to codeine rather than morphine, as suggested by Campbell et al., 2001), and not all patients benefit (as evidenced by the relatively high dropout rates owing to lack of efficacy). Intoxication and other adverse side effects appear modest and well tolerated, particularly when patients can adjust their own optimum dose. The caveats outlined earlier about the difficulty of keeping patients and their doctors "blind" to the cannabis-based medicine of course still apply to the various pain trials. There have also been few direct comparisons of Sativex (which contains equal amounts of THC and cannabidiol) with plant extracts containing THC with little or no cannabidiol, so it is difficult to assess the significance of the presence of cannabidiol, which has no significant activity at the CB-1 or CB-2 receptors.

Another common painful condition is migraine—a severe and disabling form of headache caused by local inflammation of the blood vessels in the membranes overlying the brain. Repeated migraine attacks occur in as many as 20% of women and 10% of men. During the nineteenth century cannabis was the drug of choice for the treatment of migraine (for review see Russo, 1998). But despite the earlier popularity of cannabis in the treatment of migraine, no controlled trials have as yet been described in this condition.

## Nausea and Vomiting Associated With Cancer Chemotherapy

Ironically, this condition, for which there was the earliest scientific evidence for beneficial effects of cannabis-based medicines, is now no longer seen as an area of pressing medical need—since new and even more powerful anti-sickness drugs have become available. When the cannabinoids dronabinol and nabilone were first being tested in the 1970s and early 1980s, however, matters were different. The treatment of cancer with more and more powerful drugs to suppress the growth of tumor cells advanced considerably during the 1960s and 1970s. Although the newer chemotherapy drugs were increasingly effective as anticancer agents, they brought with them severe side effects. As the British Medical Association Report (1977) put it:

> One of the most distressing symptoms in medicine is the prolonged nausea and vomiting which regularly accompanies treatment with many anti-cancer agents. This can be so severe that patients come to dread their treatment; some find the side-effects of the drugs worse than the disease they are designed to treat; others find the symptoms so intolerable that they decline further therapy despite the presence of malignant disease.

Among the most effective anticancer drugs are the platinum-containing compound cisplatin and the plant product Taxol, but unfortunately they are also very powerful in causing nausea and vomiting. Cancer patients receiving these drugs almost invariably experience nausea and vomiting, with an average of six bouts of vomiting during the first 24 hours, unless they are protected by antiemetic medicines. The initial reaction is followed by a delayed phase of nausea and vomiting during the next few days.

The results of properly controlled clinical trials conducted in the 1970s and 1980s indicated that the two cannabinoid drugs dronabinol (THC, Marinol) and nabilone appeared to offer a potentially important advance over the relatively ineffective antisickness medicines available in the early 1980s (for review see Tramer et al., 2001). The most widely used drugs then were chlorpromazine, prochlorperazine, haloperidol, metoclopramide, and domperidone—all of which act as antagonists of the chemical messenger dopamine. A total of 454 patients suffering from various forms of cancer were involved in the various clinical trials in which dronabinol was compared with placebo or with another antisickness agent, prochlorperazine. Dronabinol doses ranged from 2.5 mg/day to 40 mg/day, given as equally divided doses every 4 to 6 hours. Approximately two thirds of the patients experienced complete or partial relief from nausea and vomiting, but at the higher doses disturbing psychotropic effects were apparent in many patients (Levitt et al., 1984). The optimum dose regimen for most patients seems to be 5 mg three or four times a day (for review see British Medical Association, 1997). The use of dronabinol as an antisickness agent is supported by the results of animal experiments that show its effectiveness in various animal models, although the precise site of action in the brain remains unknown.

With nabilone, the manufacturer Eli Lilly conducted some 20 separate clinical trials involving more than 500 patients, many with a double-blind crossover design to allow the direct comparison of nabilone with prochlorperazine or other antiemetic medicines in the same patients. Nabilone proved to be as effective, or more so, as prochlorperazine and it successfully treated the symptoms of nausea and vomiting in 50% to 70% of patients. CNS side effects of drowsiness, light-headedness, and dizziness were seen in more than half of the patients, but these were not considered serious, and only a small proportion of patients (about 15%) experienced a "high" (Lemberger, 1985). The company believed that the drug could be used successfully as an antiemetic without causing intoxication, and they were successful in gaining approval from the FDA to market this product. The U.S. Drug Enforcement Agency, however, concluded that nabilone was still too much like cannabis, and they gave it a restrictive Schedule II classification; that is, it was considered to be a potentially dangerous drug of addiction, although it did have some medical usefulness. The Schedule II classification was disappointing to Eli Lilly, as it placed onerous requirements on the company and any physicians using the compound to keep it securely and to record its every movement. The company lost interest in further research in the area and did not place any major marketing effort behind nabilone, which has had little popularity.

Dronabinol and nabilone have not proved popular in clinical use. The effective dose of either cannabinoid as an antiemetic is too close to the dose that causes sedation or intoxication, and this limits the amount of drug that can be given. Patients who have not had any previous experience of exposure to cannabis generally find the psychotropic effects of the drug unpleasant and disturbing. The cannabinoids have also been eclipsed by

THE SCIENCE OF MARIJUANA

the development during the 1980s and 1990s of new and more powerful antisickness drugs. There is now a range of such medicines, some of which act by blocking one of the receptors for the chemical messenger serotonin. The 5-HT$_3$ receptor, which is targeted by these compounds, plays a key role in the neural circuits in the nervous system involved in the vomiting reflex. Another new addition has been the compound aprepitant (Emend), an antagonist of the neuropeptide substance P, which is another key player in the vomiting reflex. These new drugs have several advantages over cannabinoids. They do not suffer from the psychotropic side effects that limit the usefulness of the cannabinoid, and they are able to control nausea and vomiting in a larger proportion of patients. In addition, unlike the water-insoluble cannabinoids, they can be dissolved easily for intravenous injection. They are commonly used as an initial intravenous injection at the time of the cancer chemotherapy or radiation therapy, followed by oral tablets for the next few days. The introduction of these new drugs has radically improved cancer therapy and they have become very widely used.

## AIDS Wasting Syndrome

Loss of appetite and a progressive involuntary weight loss of about 10% of body weight are seen in AIDS wasting syndrome, a characteristic feature of the disease. The onset of bouts of wasting syndrome, which last for a month or more, is one of the defining events in the transition of HIV to AIDS. The wasting is accompanied by chronic diarrhea, weakness, and fever. The advent of the newer and more powerful treatments for HIV/AIDS may make the wasting syndrome less common in the future, but it remains a distressing feature of the disease. Although the precise physiological mechanisms underlying the wasting syndrome are not well understood, the loss of weight seems to be due primarily to reduced energy intake.

There has been considerable interest in the use of both smoked marijuana and oral dronabinol as appetite stimulants for AIDS patients. An increased appetite, particularly for sweet foods, occurring about 3 hours after smoking marijuana is well known as a feature of marijuana intoxication. Placebo-controlled studies with smoked marijuana in normal healthy volunteers have confirmed that this is a genuine phenomenon. The mechanism involved is not known, but seems to involve a combination of enhanced hunger and an increased sensory attractiveness of the foods. Repeated dosing of healthy volunteers stimulated appetite and caused a measurable increase in caloric intake.

The second approved indication for dronabinol is as an appetite stimulant to treat the loss of appetite and weight loss associated with AIDS. After a series of small-scale clinical trials gave promising results, a larger placebo-controlled clinical trial was conducted in 139 such patients (Beal et al., 1995). As compared to placebo, dronabinol treatment resulted in a statistically significant improvement in appetite after 4 or 6 weeks of treatment, and this effect persisted in those patients who continued receiving dronabinol after the end of the formal trial. There were trends toward increases in body weight and a decrease in nausea. The dose of dronabinol that appears to be optimum is 5 mg/day, administered as two doses of 2.5 mg given 1 hour before lunch and supper. Other clinical trial data suggest that dronabinol may also benefit AIDS patients suffering nausea and loss of appetite as a consequence of treatment with antiviral drugs, and some clinical studies have indicated that dronabinol causes a significant stimulation of appetite in cancer patients, who also commonly suffer loss of appetite and an accompanying body weight loss. In both cancer patients and in AIDS patients suffering from wasting syndrome the beneficial effects of dronabinol may be due in part to its ability to treat the symptoms of nausea, which often accompany these syndromes.

As in the treatment of nausea and vomiting, the principal adverse side effect in the use of dronabinol as an appetite stimulant has been the accompanying CNS side effects. While careful choice of the optimum dose and the timing of dose relative to meals can manage these in some patients, the delayed onset of action of the orally administered drug and its long duration of action are negative features.

## Other Potential Medical Targets

**Epilepsy.** Cannabis was commonly used in the nineteenth century to treat epilepsy, but there has been little interest more recently since a range of effective antiepileptic medicines became available in the twentieth century. Animal data show that THC has antiseizure activity in some experiments, but there are also conditions in which cannabinoids can make animals more susceptible to seizure activity. An interesting observation is that the nonpsychoactive cannabinoid cannabidiol was active as an antiseizure compound in some animal studies (Pertwee, 2004). There have been very few clinical studies with this compound, but one placebo-controlled trial in 15 treatment-resistant epileptic patients suggested that cannabidiol in doses of 200 or 300 mg by mouth might have beneficial effects. Cannabidiol has no appreciable activity at either of the known cannabinoid receptors, so if it is active as an anticonvulsant, this must presumably involve an action at some hitherto undiscovered cannabinoid receptor.

**Bronchial Asthma.** The possible use of cannabis in the treatment of asthma arose from studies of the effects of marijuana on respiratory function in normal healthy volunteers and in asthmatic subjects undertaken in the 1970s (Hollister, 1986). A fall of almost 40% in airway resistance was observed in volunteer studies. This led to a number of studies of smoked marijuana and oral THC in asthmatic subjects during the 1970s—a period before the modern antiasthma medicines had become available. In acute studies smoked cannabis was found to cause a bronchodilation comparable to the then standard inhalation drug isoprenaline in asthmatic subjects. However, smoked marijuana is clearly not suitable for long-term use in asthmatic subjects because of the irritant effects of various components present in the smoke. Oral THC was found to be impractical, as the doses needed for bronchodilation were clearly psychoactive. But this can be avoided by administering THC directly to the lungs by means of an aerosol. In one placebo-controlled study in 10 asthmatic subjects a THC aerosol that delivered 200µgmicrograms of THC (well below an intoxicant dose) was compared with a standard medical treatment, salbutamol aerosol (100 µg). Both drugs significantly improved respiratory function; the effect of THC was slower in onset but reached a similar maximum after 1 hour (Williams et al., 1976). However, in other studies with inhaled THC some patients found the aerosol irritating to the lung and it caused chest discomfort and cough. This inhibited further development of this line of research, although interest may be revived with the development of improved aerosol formulations (see Chapter 2).

**Mood Disorders and Sleep.** Cannabis has been advocated as a treatment for depression, anxiety, and sleep disorders. One of the first recommended uses of cannabis in Western medicine was for the treatment of depression and melancholia, and before the discovery of modern antidepressant drugs cannabis continued to be used in this way during the first half of the twentieth century. However, the few clinical trials that have been conducted with THC or nabilone in the treatment of depression or anxiety have had mixed results. Although some patients reported improvements, others found the psychic effects of the cannabinoids unpleasant and frightening. Rather than relieving anxiety, the acute effect can be to provoke anxiety and panic in some subjects—particularly those who have had no previous exposure to cannabis. Witkin et al. (2005) put forward the counterargument that the activation of CB-1 receptors on nerve terminals in the brain suppresses the release of serotonin and other monoamines thought to be important in depression, and that antagonists of CB-1 receptors might be a better approach to the treatment of depression.

In sleep laboratory studies orally administered THC at doses of 10 to 30 mg has been shown to cause increases in deep slow-wave sleep, but at the same time—as with other hypnotic drugs—there is a decrease in dreaming or rapid eye movement (REM) sleep. After repeated treatment with large doses of THC, there was evidence or some degree of hangover during the morning after treatment, and a rebound in the amount of REM sleep. THC thus does not appear to offer any advantages over existing sleeping pills, and it has the disadvantage of causing intoxication prior to sleep. Although Sativex has been found to reduce sleep disturbance in patients suffering from MS or chronic pain (see above), this is probably because it relieves the underlying symptoms leading to sleep disturbance, rather than having any direct effect on sleep mechanisms.

**Cancer.** THC and other cannabinoids have been shown to be surprisingly effective in inhibiting the proliferation of a variety of human cancer cell lines in tissue culture experiments, including breast, prostate, colorectal, gastric, lung, uterus, pancreas, and thyroid cancers (Guzman, 2005; Ligresti et al., 2006). Particularly impressive are the inhibitory effects on the growth of glioma tumors in experimental animals (Guzman, 2005). Gliomas are rapidly growing aggressive malignant cancers affecting the brain. Guzman and colleagues found that cannabinoids inhibited tumor growth by blocking the actions of factors that normally promote the growth of new blood vessels, essential for tumor growth. In a pilot clinical trial THC was injected directly into the tumors of patients with recurrent glioblastoma tumor growth, and was reported to reduce tumor cell proliferation in two of nine subjects (Guzman et al., 2006). The study of cannabinoids in cancer is in its infancy, but is potentially very interesting.

**Diarrhea.** There is a long history of the use of cannabis to control diarrhea. This is based on the presence of CB-1 receptors on the terminals of secretory nerves in the gut; activation of these receptors helps to control the overactivity of such nerves in diarrhea. Izzo and Capasso (2005) have suggested that the use of cannabis or other means of activating the cannabinoid mechanisms in the gut might represent a novel approach to the treatment of cholera, a major killer disease in the Third World.

**Emerging Indications.** Armentano (2006) reviewed recent scientific literature suggesting a potential role of cannabinoids in moderating the progression of various life-threatening diseases—in particular autoimmune disorders such as MS, rheumatoid arthritis, and inflammatory bowel disease, as well as neurodegenerative diseases such as Alzheimer disease and motoneuron disease (amyotrophic lateral sclerosis)—because of the anti-inflammatory actions of cannabinoids (Centonze et al., 2007) and their ability to counteract oxidative tissue damage. Some hints of disease-modifying actions can be seen in the clinical data from trials in MS (Zajicek et al., 2005) and in rheumatoid arthritis (Blake et al., 2006), but these are largely unexplored possibilities for the future.

## Is There Any Role for Smoked Marijuana as a Medicine?

Given the well-documented adverse effects of smoked marijuana on the lungs (see Chapter 6), is there any place at all for smoked marijuana in medicine? Apart from the potential respiratory hazards, the idea of a smoked herbal remedy goes against the grain of much of our thinking in scientifically based medicine. As the American Medical Association (1997) put it:

> The concept of burning and inhaling the combustion products of a dried plant product containing dozens of toxic and carcinogenic chemicals as a therapeutic agent represents a significant departure from the standard drug approval process. According to this viewpoint, legitimate therapeutic agents are comprised of a purified substance(s) that can be manufactured and tested in a reproducible manner.

On the other hand, there is little doubt that for many patients smoking provides a superior method of delivering THC than taking THC or cannabis extracts by mouth. Because of the variable and delayed absorption of orally administered THC, the patient is always exposed to the possibility of either under- or overdosing. Smoking, on the other hand, with some practice permits the rapid delivery of what the individual patient judges to be the correct therapeutic dose. It is clear that more research is urgently needed on alternative methods for rapidly delivering precisely gauged doses of THC, and this has been a recommendation given some priority in official reports (American Medical Association, 1997; U.S. National Institutes of Health, 1997; British Medical Association, 1997; House of Lords, Select Committee on Science and Technology, 1998; Institute of Medicine, 1999; Royal College of Physicians, 2006). The Sativex oromucosal spray (sometimes referred to as *liquid cannabis*) is a compromise between smoking and the oral route, but absorption is not particularly rapid. Some advances have been made in the development of aerosol formulations of THC and vaporizers as alternative delivery systems for cannabis (see Chapter 2), but these have not yet seen medical applications. The Canadian company

Cannasat has expressed interest in the vaporizer route of delivery, and has reported first trials of a cannabis-based medicinal product (CAT-310) in 2007 (www.cannasat.com).

A few clinical trials have attempted to assess the effectiveness of smoked marijuana, for example, in controlling the symptoms of nausea and vomiting in patients undergoing cancer chemotherapy. Some studies have used placebo marijuana cigarettes, using herbal cannabis from which THC had been extracted with alcohol beforehand. Experienced marijuana users, however, have little difficulty in distinguishing the THC-containing smoked material from the placebo, making it hard to undertake a properly blinded trial. Partly because of such difficulties, very few controlled clinical trials have ever been described (see National Institutes of Health, 1997; and American Medical Association, 1997). A recent randomized, placebo-controlled trial in 50 patients with HIV-related peripheral neuropathic pain found that smoked marijuana was more effective than placebo in pain relief (Abrams et al., 2005). This was the first controlled trial to be reported for several years.

During the late 1970s and early 1980s a number of State Departments of Health in the United States conducted open-label studies of smoked marijuana, using protocols approved by the FDA. Such studies were carried out in California, Georgia, Michigan, New Mexico, New York, and Tennessee in a total of 698 cancer patients, most of whom had not responded well to other antiemetic medicines. Unfortunately, these large studies were not well controlled; there was no attempt to use placebo, and the outcome was based not on objective measurements but on patient and/or physician ratings. Nevertheless, smoked marijuana was reported to be comparable or more effective than orally administered dronabinol and more effective than prochlorperazine or other antiemetics available at that time in reducing nausea and vomiting.

The Institute of Medicine report (1999) concluded:

There is little future in smoked marijuana as a medically approved medication.

But despite this, smoked marijuana is used illegally by thousands of people, and it is permitted for medical use in 12 states in the United States, where more than 100,000 patients are registered users. In the Netherlands the medical use of cannabis was legalized in 2003, so physicians can prescribe herbal cannabis to patients through pharmacies that supply medical-grade cannabis. The most common indications are for the treatment of pain associated with neurological disease (e.g., MS) or rheumatoid arthritis and for loss of appetite associated with cancer. A survey showed that almost two thirds of patients reported good or excellent effects on their symptoms, and side effects were generally mild (Gorter et al., 2005). In Canada, the law was relaxed in 2003 to allow the cultivation and supply of medicinal cannabis. Patients are supplied cannabis by Health Canada on prescription, and a company, Amigula Inc., has been formed to provide standardized medical-grade herbal cannabis and low-tar resin (http://www.amigula.com).

## A Cannabinoid Antagonist for the Treatment of Obesity

The involvement of cannabinoid mechanisms in the control of food intake and body weight has already been referred to. The discovery that the antagonist rimonabant was capable of blocking these mechanisms both in the brain and in the periphery prompted clinical trials of this drug in the treatment of obesity, and the positive results of these trials led to its approval in Europe in 2006 as a potentially important new medicine for combating the ever-increasing problem of obesity in Western societies. The history of the rapid development of rimonabant since the first scientific publication in 1994 (Rinaldi-Carmona et al., 1994) is a good example of how preclinical data can suggest and guide a clinical development program (reviewed by Carai et al., 2006).

### Preclinical Data

A number of studies showed that rimonabant caused a marked reduction in daily food intake when given to normal or obese rats and mice given unlimited access to normal or high-fat diets. It was particularly effective in reducing the intake of palatable foods—normally consumed avidly even by satiated rats (e.g., condensed milk, chocolate-flavored drinks). This was accompanied by significant reductions in body weight. However, the effects of rimonabant on food intake diminished with repeated dosing, and were no longer seen after the first week. Despite this, the drug continued to cause reductions in body weight, even though food intake had recovered to near-normal levels. This could be explained by the finding of increased energy expenditure in the treated animals. A key target seems to be the fat tissue, whose cells carry CB-1 receptors. Blockade of these receptors led to increased synthesis and release into the circulation of the hormone adiponectin, which plays an important role in energy balance. Adiponectin stimulates the metabolism of fatty acids (otherwise deposited as fat), decreases plasma glucose levels, and decreases body weight. CB-1 receptors in the liver may also be involved, as activation of these receptors stimulates fatty acid synthesis and promotes diet-induced obesity (Osei-Hyiaman et al., 2005). Rimonabant treatment of animals made obese by overfeeding showed decreased amounts of fat tissue, increased energy expenditure and fat breakdown; normalized plasma levels of glucose; reductions in plasma levels of triglycerides (fat); decreases in bad, low-density lipoprotein (LDL) cholesterol; and decreases in the otherwise abnormally high amounts of another key hormone, leptin, in plasma. Leptin is made by fat cells and secreted into the circulation. In the brain it acts on the hypothalamus to cause a reduction in food intake, as part of the complex mechanisms whereby the brain helps to control food intake and body weight (Morton et al., 2006). These findings from animal experiments formed a valuable translational bridge to guide the subsequent clinical studies.

Clinical Data

The results of three large-scale randomized double-blind placebo-controlled clinical trials have been reported, involving a total of 5,584 patients in Europe and the United States (reviewed by Carai et al., 2006). All three trials involved daily treatment with 5 or 20 mg rimonabant or placebo for 1 year. Subjects were overweight or obese and in addition to drug treatment agreed to observe a calorie-restricted diet. A variety of weight and other outcome measures were evaluated. In one of the trials treatment was continued (or discontinued) for a further period of 1 year.

The results were remarkable. All three studies yielded very similar data—in terms of weight loss after 1 year, patients receiving 20 mg rimonabant lost 6.3 to 6.9 kg, compared to a loss of 1.5 to 1.8 kg in the placebo groups (Fig. 5.4). The weight loss was accompanied by significant decreases in waist circumference—showing that the drug was particularly effective in reducing abdominal fat—known to be a risk factor for cardiovascular disease. In addition, rimonabant caused significant decreases in plasma glucose and fat levels; increases in plasma levels of adiponectin; reduced levels of leptin; and elevations in good, high-density lipoprotein (HDL) cholesterol—indicating protective effects against a number of known risk factors for heart disease. Patients maintained on rimonabant for a second year maintained the reduction in body weight and improved metabolic parameters.

As might be expected in large-scale trials with demanding requirements (e.g., calorie-reduced diet), a significant proportion of the patients in each trial dropped out before completing the trial (40% to 50%), but there were no differences in dropout rates between drug-treated and placebo groups. A variety of adverse events were reported by subjects, but most of these did not differ between placebo and treated groups. Rimonabant appears to be well tolerated and safe; the only side effects seen more frequently in patients receiving 20 mg rimonabant were episodes of dizziness, nausea, anxiety, and depression—but these occurred at low frequencies and did not seem to be major reasons for patients dropping out of the trials. The low incidence of depression/anxiety in response to blockade of CB-1 receptors by rimonabant is remarkable, given the euphoriant effects that cannabis has—perhaps this tells us that the cannabinoid system in the brain is not normally very active, and may be called into intense activity only in conditions such as stress.

It is likely that rimonabant will find a place in the treatment of obesity-related disorders, and these will include diabetes, which is associated with obesity, and the metabolic syndrome described previously. Positive results from a controlled clinical trial of rimonabant in patients with type 2 diabetes were reported in 2006, and showed improved control of plasma

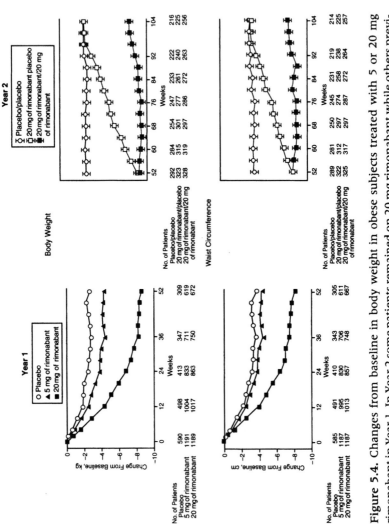

**Figure 5.4.** Changes from baseline in body weight in obese subjects treated with 5 or 20 mg rimonabant in Year 1. In Year 2 some patients remained on 20 mg rimonabant while others previously treated with this dose were switched to placebo. (*JAMA* 2006; 295:768. Copyright © 2006, American Medical Association. All rights reserved.)

glucose, reduced body weight, and improvements in the metabolic parameters previously described.

Critics of rimonabant have pointed out that the drug does not continue to reduce body weight after the first few months of treatment (Fig. 5.4)—and a loss of 6 to 7 kg may not amount to that much for someone who may weigh 150 kg or more. The results from patients who discontinued rimonabant treatment showed that body weight climbed gradually back to initial baseline levels after 12 months (Fig. 5.4). Furthermore, the clinical trial data, although impressive, only refer to the patients who completed the trials. Only those subjects who showed themselves capable of adhering to the calorie-controlled diet in a 1-month run-up period were admitted to the studies, and even so, 40% dropped out before completing. Nevertheless, some have predicted that rimonabant could be the next "blockbuster" in the pharmaceutical world, and many other companies are racing to provide their own CB-1 antagonist medicines—more than six such products are in clinical trials currently.

However, although rimonabant was approved in 2006 as a prescription medicine in Europe, its future in the United States suffered a major setback in June 2007, when expert advisers to the FDA recommended against its approval in the United States, citing the small but worrying instance of adverse psychiatric side effects, including anxiety, depression, sleep disorders, and an increased tendency to suicidality. European regulators have also sought a reappraisal of the rimonabant safety profile.

## Conclusions

There are clearly several possible therapeutic indications for cannabis-based medicines, but for many of them evidence for the clinical effectiveness of the drug is still inadequate by modern standards. This situation has improved in recent years, however, as new data from controlled clinical trials became available. One of the obvious complications in the medical use of cannabis is that the window between its therapeutic effects and the cannabis-induced high is often narrow. As the Institute of Medicine (1999) report points out, however, this can sometimes be beneficial to the patient.

Older patients with no previous experience of cannabis may find the psychic effects of the drug disturbing and unpleasant. But in some conditions the antianxiety effects of cannabis can have a beneficial effect, since anxiety itself tends to make the symptoms worse (e.g., in movement disorders, cancer chemotherapy, and AIDS wasting syndrome).

The other requirement for a human medicine is that it should be safe to use, and the next chapter will address that question.

# 6

## *Is Cannabis Safe?*

The initial enthusiasm for cannabis in the 1960s and early 1970s was rapidly followed by a wave of reaction in the Western world. Many parents were appalled that their children were taking this relatively unknown drug and feared that it might damage their health or impair their education. Although scientists are supposed to try to minimize bias, this has been difficult to avoid in a field so colored by issues of morality and public policy, and some have been guided by a moral commitment to prove that cannabis is harmful. Extravagant warnings were given, suggesting that cannabis was a highly dangerous drug that could cause chromosomal damage, impotence, sterility, respiratory damage, depressed immune system responses, personality changes, and permanent brain damage. Most of these claims were later proved to be spurious and the balanced reviews by Hollister (1986, 1998) and by L. Zimmer and J.P. Morgan (1997), in their entertaining book *Marijuana Myths, Marijuana Facts*, showed how effectively many of them could be demolished. It is thus not necessary to deal with all of these arguments in detail here, but simply to highlight some of the factors that may determine whether cannabis is considered sufficiently safe to be reintroduced into Western medicine and ultimately whether its overall prohibition remains justified.

## Toxicity

THC is a very safe drug. Laboratory animals (rats, mice, dogs, monkeys) can tolerate doses of up to 1,000 mg/kg. This would be equivalent to a 70-kg person swallowing 70 g of the drug—about 5,000 times more than is required to produce a high. Despite the widespread illicit use of cannabis, there are very few if any instances of people dying from an overdose. In Britain, the National Statistics Office listed no deaths related to cannabis in the period 2000–2004, while there were estimated to be 3 million cannabis users. By comparison with other commonly used recreational drugs, these statistics are impressive. In Britain, there are some 1,000 deaths due to heroin or other opiate overdose, more than 100,000 alcohol-related deaths, and at least as many tobacco-related deaths each year (Advisory Council on Misuse of Drugs, 2006). Even such apparently innocuous medicines as aspirin and related nonsteroidal anti-inflammatory compounds are not safe. It has been estimated that more than 7,000 Americans die every year because of the tendency of these drugs to cause catastrophic gastric bleeding (Fries, 1992). Hundreds more die while taking the painkiller paracetamol, because of its tendency to cause liver damage.

Long-term toxicology studies with THC were sponsored by the National Institute of Mental Health in the late 1960s (Braude, 1972). These included a 90-day study with a 30-day recovery period in both rats and monkeys. These studies were similar in design to those required for any new medicine before it can be approved for human use. Large numbers of animals were exposed to high doses of the drug every day, and blood samples were taken regularly to look for biochemical abnormalities during the study. At the end of the study a careful autopsy was performed on each animal, recording the weight and appearance of internal organs. Sections of the major organs were subsequently examined under the microscope to look for any pathological changes. Interestingly, these studies included not only delta-9-tetrahydrocannabinol (THC) but also delta-8-THC and a crude extract of marijuana. Treatment of animals with doses of cannabis or cannabinoids in the range of 50 to 500 mg/kg led to decreased food intake and lower body weight. All three test substances initially depressed behavior but later animals became more active, and were irritable or aggressive. At the end of the study decreased organ weights were seen in the ovary, uterus, prostate, and spleen and increases were seen in the adrenals. The behavioral and organ changes were similar in monkeys but less severe than those seen in rats. Further studies were carried out to assess the potential damage that might be done to the developing fetus by exposure to cannabis or cannabinoids during pregnancy. Treatment of pregnant rabbits with THC at doses of up to 5 mg/kg had no effect on birth weight and did not cause any abnormalities in the offspring. Dr. Braude concluded:

> In summary, I would like to say that Delta-9-THC given orally seems to be a rather safe compound in animals as well as in man and appears to have little teratological potential even at dose levels considerably higher than the typical human dose.

Chan et al. (1996) reported the findings of similarly detailed toxicology studies carried out with THC by the National Institute of Environmental Health Sciences in the United States, in response to a request from the National Cancer Institute. Groups of rats and mice were treated repeatedly with a range of doses of THC dissolved in corn oil, including doses many times higher than those likely to be used clinically. Each dose of the drug was administered to a separate group of 10 male and 10 female animals. In both species the doses ranged from 0 to 500 mg/kg. The animals were treated five times a week for 13 weeks, and some groups of animals were followed for a further period of 9 weeks' recovery. By the end of the study more than half of the rats treated with the highest dose (500 mg/kg) had died, but all of the remaining animals appeared healthy, although in both species the higher doses caused lethargy and increased aggressiveness. The THC-treated animals ate less food and their body weights were consequently significantly lower than those of untreated controls at the end of the treatment period, but they rose back to normal levels during the subsequent recovery period. During this period animals were sensitive to touch and some exhibited convulsions. There was a tendency for the drug to cause decreases in the weight of the uterus and testes.

In further studies groups of rats were treated with doses of THC up to 50 mg/kg and mice with up to 500 mg/kg, five times a week for 2 years, a standard test to determine whether new medical compounds were liable to cause cancers. At the end of the 2 years more treated animals had survived than controls—probably because the treated animals ate less and had lower body weights. The treated animals also showed a significantly *lower* incidence of the various cancers normally seen in aged rodents, in the testes, pancreas, pituitary gland, mammary gland, liver, and uterus. Although there was an increased incidence of precancerous changes in the thyroid gland in both species and in the mouse ovary after one dose (125 mg/kg), these changes were not dose related. The conclusion was that there was "no evidence of carcinogenic activity of THC at doses up to 50 mg/kg." This was also supported by the failure to detect any genetic toxicity in other tests designed to identify drugs capable of causing chromosomal damage. For example, THC was negative in the so-called Ames test in which bacteria are exposed to very high concentrations of the test drug to see whether it induces any mutations. In another standard test hamster ovary cells were exposed to high concentrations of the drug in tissue culture, and no effects were observed on cell division that might indicate chromosomal damage.

There have been claims that chronic cannabis use may permanently damage the brain, but there is little scientific evidence to support this (for reviews see Zimmer and Morgan, 1997; and Hollister, 1986, 1998). The earlier studies have been complemented by the application of powerful modern neuroimaging methods. For example, a magnetic resonance imaging (MRI) study compared 18 current, frequent, young adult cannabis users with 13 comparable nonusers and found no evidence of cerebral atrophy or regional changes in tissue volumes (Block et al., 2000).

Animal studies have yielded conflicting results (for review see Iversen, 2003). Although some studies have reported hippocampal damage in rats exposed to high doses of THC, the 2-year carcinogenicity studies referred to previously (Chan et al., 1998) failed to find any pathological changes in the brains of rats or mice after long-term exposure to very high doses. Although claims were made that exposure of a small number of rhesus monkeys to cannabis smoke led to ultrastructural changes in the septum and hippocampus (Harper et al., 1977; Heath et al., 1980), subsequent larger scale studies failed to show any cannabis-induced histopathology in monkey brain (Scallet, 1991).

Studies of the effects of cannabinoids on neurons in tissue culture have also yielded inconsistent results. Exposure of rat cortical neurons to THC was reported to decrease their survival, with twice as many cells dead after a 2-hour exposure to 5 μM THC than in control cultures (Downer et al., 2001). Toxic effects of THC have also been reported on hippocampal neurons in culture, with 50% cell death after 2 hours' exposure to 10 μM THC or after 5 days' exposure to 1 μM drug (Chan et al., 1998). The antagonist rimonabant blocked these effects. On the other hand, other authors failed to observe any damage in rat cortical neurones exposed for up to 15 days to 1 μM THC (Sánchez et al., 1998).

Some studies have even reported neuroprotective actions of cannabinoids. Administration of WIN55,212-2 was found to reduce cerebral damage in rat hippocampus or cerebral cortex in an animal model of stroke (Nagayama et al., 1999), and rat hippocampal neurons in tissue culture were protected again glutamate-mediated damage by low concentrations of WIN55,212–2 or CP55,940; these effects were again mediated through CB-1 receptors (Shen and Thayer, 1998). The mixed reports of neurotoxic and neuroprotective effects of cannabinoids are confusing. While it may be possible to demonstrate neurotoxic actions after exposure of neurons to high concentrations of cannabinoids in vitro, there is little evidence for any significant neural damage in vivo after the administration of pharmacologically relevant doses of these drugs. By any standards, THC must be considered to be a very safe drug both acutely and on long-term exposure. The very low lethality of the drug may reflect the fact that cannabinoid receptors are virtually absent from those regions at the base of the brain that are responsible for such vital functions as breathing and blood pressure control. The available animal data are more than adequate to justify its approval as a human medicine, and indeed it has been approved by the Food and Drug Administration (FDA) for certain limited therapeutic indications.

## Acute Effects of Cannabis

Of all the immediate actions of cannabis (Chapters 2 and 3), its psychoactive effects are undoubtedly those that give the greatest concern in considering the medical uses of the drug. In several of the medical applications that have been assessed to date, unwanted psychic side effects have been cited as the main reason for patients rejecting the drug as unacceptable. Patients who have had no prior experience with cannabis often find the intoxicant effects disturbing and the drug may induce a frightening panic/anxiety attack in such people. Others may simply not want to be high when they go about their daily work. The deleterious effects of cannabis on short-term memory and other aspects of cognition (Chapter 4) make it especially unacceptable for those whose occupation depends on an ability to remain alert and capable of handling and processing complex information. If improved delivery systems could be devised, it is more likely that patients could self-adjust their optimum doses of the drug to avoid some of these unwanted effects, but it appears that the therapeutic window between a medically effective dose and an intoxicant one is narrow. A more serious acute reaction is a form of toxic psychosis. The symptoms can be severe enough to lead to admission to emergency psychiatric wards. In some of the psychiatric literature this is referred to as *cannabis psychosis* (or *marijuana psychosis*) (Thomas, 1993; Johns, 2001; Castle and Murray, 2004). It nearly always results from taking large doses of the drug, often in food or drink, and the condition may persist for some days. The initial diagnosis can be confused with schizophrenia, since the patients may display some of the characteristic symptoms of schizophrenic illness. These include delusions of control (being under the control of some outside being or force), grandiose identity, persecution, thought insertion, auditory hallucinations (hearing sounds, usually nonverbal in nature), changed perception, and blunting of the emotions. Not all symptoms will be seen in every patient, but there is a considerable similarity to paranoid schizophrenia. This has lead some to propose a cannabinoid hypothesis of schizophrenia, suggesting that the symptoms of schizophrenic illness might be caused by an abnormal overactivity of endogenous cannabinoid mechanisms in the brain (Emrich et al., 1997). D'Souza et al. (2004) developed a model for studying cannabis psychosis under laboratory conditions; schizophrenia-like psychotic symptoms could be induced in healthy volunteers within a few minutes following the intravenous injection of THC, and these symptoms persisted for 1 to 2 hours. Cannabis is not unique in sometimes causing acute psychotic reactions. Similar effects are commonly seen with amphetamines, cocaine, ketamine, phencyclidine, and alcohol (Thirthalli and Benegal, 2006).

Along with these psychic effects go impairments in psychomotor skills, so that for a period of some hours after taking the drug it is inadvisable to drive, and the ability of users to carry out any tasks that require manual dexterity is likely to be impaired (Chapter 4). A drug-induced impairment of balance could also make elderly patients more likely to fall. A comparison of 452 marijuana smokers with a similar number of nonsmokers attending the Kaiser Permanente health group in California revealed that the marijuana smokers had an increased risk of attending outpatient clinics with injuries of various types—perhaps as a result of the acute intoxicant effects of the drug (Polen et al., 1993).

There are also quite profound effects of cannabis on the heart and vascular system (Chapter 2). In inexperienced users the drug can cause a large increase in heart rate (up to a doubling) and this could be harmful to someone with a previous history of coronary artery disease or heart failure. Such patients should be excluded from any clinical trials of cannabis-based medicines for this reason. The postural hypotension that can be caused by cannabis could also be distressing or possibly dangerous, as the fall in blood pressure when rising from a seated or lying down position can result in fainting. The effects of the drug on the cardiovascular system usually show rapid tolerance on repeated exposure to cannabis, so for normal healthy subjects these effects do not appear to be of any particular concern.

## Effects of Long-Term Exposure to Cannabis

### Are There Persistent Cognitive Deficits?

The acute effects of marijuana on working memory are relatively short lived, and disappear after 3 to 4 hours as the marijuana high wears off. Considerable attention has been paid to the possibility that there might be more persistent effects of marijuana on intellectual function, in particular, whether people who regularly use large doses of marijuana suffer any long-term cognitive impairment. Because of the political implications for marijuana policy, the interpretation of the results of such studies has long been controversial and different studies have sometimes reached apparently divergent conclusions. Fortunately, there have been several excellent reviews of this confusing literature, which help to understand it. Van Amsterdam et al. (1996) and Earleywine (2002) point out the many methodological difficulties inherent in studies of the long-term consequences of marijuana use. Among the confounding factors in human studies are that comparisons have to be made between groups of drug users versus nonusers; it is usually impossible to compare the baseline performance of these groups prior to cannabis use to see if they are properly matched. How does one ensure that the results from a group of chronic drug users are compared with a suitable control group of nondrug users, matched for age, educational attainment, and other demographic factors? Statistical analysis of such data has often been poor—common errors being to use so many different tests that the likelihood of finding some significant differences is increased or the use of inadequate sample sizes. When should the drug users be tested? Most studies have been done in a period of 12 to 48 hours after last drug use, but the results may simply reflect a residual effect of the drug or the withdrawal symptoms that heavy users suffer from when they stop taking marijuana, which could also impair their cognitive performance during the immediate period after drug cessation. Pope et al. (2001), for example, recruited 63 current heavy users who had smoked cannabis at least 5,000 times in their lives and 72 control subjects. Subjects underwent a 28-day washout from cannabis use, monitored by urine assays. At days 0, 1, and 7 of the abstinence period the heavy users scored significantly below control subjects on a battery of neuropsychological tests, particularly in recall of word lists. However, by day 28 there were virtually no differences between the groups on any of the test results, and there was no significant association between cumulative lifetime cannabis use and test scores. Many of the published studies suffer so severely from such limitations that their conclusions are equivocal at best. Most recent analyses of the literature have concluded that there are indeed significant residual drug effects in the period 12 to 24 hours after last drug use, and these can be observed in various tests of psychomotor function, attention, and short-term memory. The evidence for any more persistent cognitive deficits is equivocal. Although persistent impairments in various cognitive tests have been reported, these are not consistent from one study to another.

During the 1970s the National Institute for Drug Abuse commissioned a series of detailed studies of long-term marijuana users in countries in which heavy use of the drug is endemic. A series of carefully conducted studies were performed, for example, in Costa Rica, which has a literate Westernized culture (Satz et al., 1976). Several studies during the 1970s and 1980s compared frequent marijuana users with nonusers using a battery of anthropological and neuropsychological tests, but failed to find any significant differences. It was only in a follow-up study reported in 1996 that any significant cognitive differences were found in a cohort of 17 older marijuana users (aged older than 45 years). These men had consumed marijuana on average for 34 years, smoking about five joints per day. They were tested after a 72-hour period of abstinence using an impressive array of cognitive tasks designed to investigate various aspects of memory and attention. Statistically significant deficits were observed in only a few of the more complex verbal memory tasks, and these differences were relatively small (<10% impairment relative to controls). The same battery of tests applied to a younger group of heavy marijuana users failed to reveal any significant deficits. The authors concluded that:

> ... The deficiencies observed in this study ... are subtle. The older long-term users are largely functional and employable, and they do not demonstrate the types of dementia and amnesic syndromes associated with alcohol use of comparable magnitude. (Fletcher et al., 1996)

Similar studies of long-term heavy users in Jamaica (Bowman and Pihl, 1973) and Greece, countries in which heavy marijuana use is endemic, failed to reveal any notable differences in cognitive function between marijuana users and nonusers. The U.S. National Institute of Mental Health commissioned a number of scientific studies to assess the effects of prolonged heavy consumption of cannabis in Jamaica. Comparisons of heavy smokers with nonsmokers revealed surprisingly few adverse effects of smoking on physical health or work performance. In a particularly famous study, Comitas (1976) reported data that seemed to refute the then popular belief that cannabis consumption led to an *amotivational syndrome*. On the contrary:

> As reflected in their verbal responses, the belief and attitudes of lower class users about ganja and work are not at all ambiguous. Ganja is universally perceived as an energizer, a motive power—never as an enervator that leads to apathy and immobility. In Jamaica, ganja, at least on the ideational level, permits its users to face, start and carry out the most difficult and distasteful manual labor. (Comitas, 1976)

Comitas went on to show by objective measurements that the productivity of sugar cane cutters was no different when ganja smokers were compared with nonsmokers.

Nevertheless, while this may be true for gross deficits in function, many would now agree that long-term marijuana use can lead to subtle and selective impairments in cognitive function. This area of research has been a particular interest of Nadia Solowij, and her monograph *Cannabis and Cognitive Functioning* (Solowij, 1998) gives an excellent review. Subtle cognitive impairments can be observed in ex-marijuana smokers in tests that measure the ability to organize and integrate complex information, sometimes described as *executive function*. The size of the deficit is related to the frequency of marijuana consumption and the duration. In addition to deficits in subtle neuropsychological tests, Solowij described abnormalities in "event-related potentials" in ex-marijuana smokers. These are small electrical discharges that can be recorded from the scalp in response to auditory stimuli that require the subject to make a decision and take some action. The results suggested that subjects were unable to reject complex irrelevant information and hence were less able to focus their attention effectively. In other words, they suffered from a defect in selective attention, a process that is necessary for the successful completion of most cognitive tasks. Although these deficits may not have much impact on the ability of ex-marijuana smokers to function normally, they add further weight to the conclusion that marijuana tends to impair executive function in the brain.

In summary, although there have been many rumors that the long-term use of marijuana leads to irreversible damage to higher brain functions, the results of numerous scientific studies have failed to confirm this. The report to the Dutch government prepared by van Amsterdam et al. (1996) sums this up as follows:

> In all studies complete matching of users and non-users was only partly accomplished and the time between cannabis use and testing (duration of abstinence) was too short to ascertain absence of drug residues in the body. Based on the results of the three best studies performed (Schwartz, Pope and Block et al) residual cognitive effects are seldom observed and if present they are mild in nature.

## Tolerance and Dependence

As described in Chapter 4, there is a growing recognition that both tolerance and dependence do occur in some people, perhaps in as many as 10% of regular cannabis users (discussed in more detail in Chapter 7). Tolerance to some of the unwanted effects of the drug on the cardiovascular system or to the unpleasant psychic effects may be regarded as positive features, but the possibility of becoming psychologically dependent on the drug is a matter for genuine concern. For some people the drug may come to dominate their lives, and in extreme cases lead to a semipermanent state of intoxication. How important an issue this is in considering the medical use of cannabis remains unclear. Among illicit users of cannabis it seems that only those who regularly consume large amounts of the drug are at risk of becoming dependent. The medical users of the drug usually take relatively small doses of cannabis on an intermittent basis and are, therefore, much less likely to become dependent. Case reports from individual patients often stress that they do not want to become high, and that they use the drug only occasionally. Data from the controlled trials of Sativex show that even when treated for 2 years or more, patients did not increase the dose used, which remained surprisingly constant (Chapter 5).

## Adverse Effects on Fertility and the Unborn Child

A paper published in the prestigious *New England Journal of Medicine* in 1974 sounded alarm bells (Kolodny et al., 1974). The authors reported that blood levels of the male hormone testosterone were severely depressed (average 56% of normal) in 20 young men who were regular marijuana users. In addition, some of the subjects were reported to have reduced sperm counts. These findings, of course, raised immediate concerns about the possibility that marijuana use might impair male sexual function or even lead to sterility and impotence. Numerous follow-up studies, however, either failed to repeat the original findings or found milder changes in testosterone levels or spermatogenesis (Zimmer and Morgan, 1997). Less research has been done in women, although there have been some reports of menstrual cycle abnormalities and transient reductions in prolactin levels. There is little evidence for long-term infertility associated with marijuana use in humans; nor is there evidence of reduced fertility in those countries where heavy use of cannabis is endemic (Zimmer and Morgan, 1997).

Changes in the secretion of sex hormones are presumably mediated by actions of cannabis in the hypothalamus, which controls such secretions. But CB-1 receptors are also present in quite high density in the testes and uterus and on preimplantation human embryos. One hypothesis is that endogenous cannabinoids may be involved in regulating early embryonic development, perhaps influencing the window of implantation of the blastocyst in the uterus (Wang et al., 2006). As described earlier (Chapter 3), a delicate balance of endocannabinoid mechanisms in the human blastocyst and uterus may determine the likelihood of a successful embryo implantation. Heavy use of cannabis has been associated with a temporary reduction in fertility and early miscarriage (Paria and Dey, 2000; Maccarrone and Finazzi-Agrò, 2004; Wang et al., 2006). A number of studies in animals have also shown that THC can cause spontaneous abortions, low birth weight, and physical deformities—but these were generally seen only after treatment with very high doses of THC (Paria and Dey, 2000).

Several studies have compared the babies born to women who had used marijuana during pregnancy with the babies of women who did not. Many studies failed to show any significant differences, but there is a consistent tendency toward a shorter gestation period and smaller birth weight in babies born to mothers who used marijuana. However, although a significantly lower birth weight was observed in the largest such study (involving 12,424 births), when other factors were taken into account (e.g., tobacco smoking), there was no statistically meaningful relation between marijuana use and low birth weight (Zuckerman et al., 1989). Similarly, a trend toward a higher incidence of birth abnormalities in the marijuana-exposed group in the same study was also not considered statistically meaningful. If marijuana smoking does cause a reduction in birth weight, this is quite likely to be due to the presence of carbon monoxide in marijuana smoke. This gas binds tightly to the red pigment hemoglobin in the blood, making it less able to carry oxygen to the growing fetus. It is thought that the carbon monoxide in cigarette smoke is the most likely factor to account for the well-documented effect of tobacco smoking during pregnancy on reduced birth weight.

Several studies examined the development of children born to mothers who were exposed to marijuana during pregnancy, to see whether any abnormalities in physical or mental development could be detected. While the results of the majority of these investigations were negative, the few instances in which subtle abnormalities could be detected in subsets of the IQ scale have been used as evidence that marijuana can impair children's cognitive development. In one of the largest studies of this kind, psychologist Peter Fried and colleagues examined a group of more than 100 children whose mothers were exposed to marijuana. In his Ottawa Prenatal Prospective Study hundreds of different psychological tests were administered to the children, but very few differences were found between the marijuana-exposed versus nonexposed groups. But when the children were 6 years old, subtle deficits in frontal lobe executive functions were reported, involving visual memory, analysis, and integration, and these persisted when the children were examined again at age 13 to 16 years (Fried et al., 2003). But a further study of the cohort at age 18 to 22, using brain imaging and cognitive tests, failed to detect deficits in working memory (Smith et al., 2006). The differences noted in the babies born to mothers who used marijuana were relatively minor by comparison with the consistent cognitive deficits observed in children of all ages born to mothers who had been heavy cigarette smokers during pregnancy (Fried, 1993). (For reviews see Maccarrone and Wenger, 2005; and Wang et al., 2006.)

### Suppression of Immune System Function

Reports during the 1970s seemed at first to provide alarming evidence of a suppression of normal immune system function in chronic marijuana users. Nahas et al. (1974), for example, claimed that white blood cells of the T-cell type isolated from marijuana users and incubated in tissue culture did not show the normal growth and transformation responses when challenged with immune system stimulants. Other reports suggested that T-lymphocytes might be reduced in numbers in marijuana smokers. But the initial reports were not confirmed by subsequent studies, and most would now question the validity of the earlier claims (Zimmer and Morgan, 1997).

Nevertheless, the discovery that the second cannabinoid receptor CB-2 is located principally on the various cell types of the immune system, the macrophages, T-cells, B-cells, and mast cells, has renewed interest in the interaction of cannabinoids with the immune system. Studies in animals confirmed that treatment with high doses of THC was immunosuppressant. Treated animals were more susceptible to viral or bacterial infections and showed impaired tissue rejection responses, for example, to skin transplants. There has been interest by pharmaceutical companies in developing CB-2–selective drugs, which might have utility as immunosuppressants or in the treatment of such diseases as arthritis or multiple sclerosis, which are thought to be due to inappropriate immune system responses. CB-2 knockout mice, which are genetically engineered to prevent expression of CB-2 receptors, however, exhibit largely unimpaired immune system function, although there may be defects in the development of the B- and T-cell subsets (Ziring et al., 2006).

Despite the evidence for suppression of immune system function in animals, there is no evidence that the long-term recreational or medical use of cannabis renders users more susceptible to bacterial or viral infection (Cabral and Staab, 2005). Patients suffering from HIV infection might be expected to be at particular risk, since their immune systems are already impaired as a result of the viral infection. However, longitudinal studies involving several thousands of such patients have failed to show any effect of marijuana use on the progression of the disease to full-blown AIDS (Kaslow et al., 1989; Cabral and Staab, 2005). (For review see Cabral and Staab, 2005.)

Cannabis and Mental Illness

The concern that the use of cannabis might precipitate mental illness in some users is a long-standing one. There was a lively correspondence in the columns of the *British Medical Journal* in 1893, for example, as to whether or not the endemic use of hashish in Egypt led to mania and insanity (*BMJ*, 1893, pp. 710, 813, 920, 969, 1027). There was concern that the mental asylums in British India were filling with cannabis-induced lunatics, and this was one of the factors that led the British government to appoint the Indian Hemp Drugs Commission (1894) (see Chapter 8). The Commission undertook a large and painstaking review and concluded that there were virtually no patients in the Indian asylums whose illness could be attributed to cannabis use. The Commission's findings were not widely noted, however, and claims of a relationship between cannabis use and insanity continued to be made in India and in many other countries. Claims that cannabis use leads to insanity were used by early advocates of marijuana prohibition in the United States. In recent years this debate has been reopened by the publication of a number of studies that show an association between teenage cannabis use and the development of psychotic symptoms in adulthood. Academic psychiatrists in Britain called on the government to reconsider the downgrading in the legal status of cannabis in light of these findings (see Chapter 8).

A number of studies have addressed the contentious question of whether cannabis use can precipitate long-term psychiatric illness. The strongest evidence came from a study in Sweden, which involved taking detailed medical records and information about the social background and drug-taking habits of more than 50,000 conscripts on entry to the Swedish army at age 18 to 20 (1969–1970) and following up their subsequent medical history over a 15-year period (Andreasson et al., 1987, 1989). A total of 5,391 of the conscripts admitted having taken cannabis at least once, but the cannabis users accounted for a disproportionate number of the 246 cases of schizophrenic illness diagnosed in the overall group on follow-up. The relative risk of schizophrenia in those who had used cannabis was 2.4 times greater than in the nonusers. And in the small number of heavy users (who had taken the drug on more than 50 occasions), the relative risk of schizophrenia increased to 6.0. The authors concluded that cannabis was an independent risk factor for schizophrenia. Six other similar reports involving smaller numbers of subjects were published subsequently and all reached the same conclusion (reviewed by Arseneault et al., 2004; Semple et al., 2005; Henquet et al., 2005). Moore et al. (2007) pooled the data from all of these studies and concluded that the overall odds ratio linking cannabis use to subsequent psychosis was 1.4; that is, cannabis use was associated with a 40% increased risk of developing a schizophrenia-like psychosis in later life. At first sight these findings seem convincing and alarming, but they do not necessarily prove that a cause-and-effect relationship exists between cannabis and psychosis.

The problem with studies of this type is that the association may be related to some common predisposing factor (known as a confounding factor); these might include personality, tendency to psychotic thought processes, gender, family background, use of other drugs, etc. Indeed, some psychologists and psychiatrists believe that they can identify psychological traits, which are described as *schizotypy* and which may predict an increased risk of developing clinical psychosis. Some studies in healthy adults have reported that those subjects who used cannabis scored higher on schizotypy scales than nonusers (Williams et al., 1996). Such findings would support a reverse causality theory—that is, that pre-existing psychotic symptoms in teenagers might predispose them toward cannabis use. However, several of the modern studies have taken this into account as an important confounding factor, but significant associations remain, although odds ratios are reduced by excluding this factor. Another problem is multidrug use. Half of the cannabis-using subjects in the original Swedish study who had used cannabis more than 10 times and subsequently developed schizophrenia had also taken amphetamine—a drug known to be capable of inducing a schizophrenia-like psychosis. The cannabis users also came from deprived social backgrounds, another known risk factor of schizophrenia. A more detailed follow-up of the data from the original Swedish cohort attempted to take into account some of these confounding factors (Zammit et al., 2002). The result was to reduce the odds ratios considerably, although there was still a significant association between cannabis use and psychosis, apparently dose-related (Table 6.1). Others attempted a rigorous mathematical analysis that would take into account even unidentified confounding factors and still found a significant association (Fergusson et al., 2005). An interesting idea is that genetic factors may increase the risk of psychosis developing in cannabis users. Caspi et al. (2005) reported that carriers of a particular genetic form of the enzyme catechol-O-methyl transferase (COMT), which is involved in inactivating dopamine in the brain, were more likely to develop psychosis in later life following teenage cannabis use than carriers of another genetic form of the enzyme. Although the numbers of subjects involved were very small, this is an intriguing possibility. Can we envisage the possibility of the genetic screening of young people in the future to determine whether it is safe for them to use cannabis?

Table 6.1. Crude and Adjusted Odds Ratios for Developing Schizophrenia in Swedish Conscripts Cohort

| Drug Use | No. of Subjects | No. Developing Schizophrenia | Crude Odds Ratio | Adjusted Odds Ratio* |
|---|---|---|---|---|
| No cannabis ever | 36,429 | 215 | 1.0 | 1.0 |
| Cannabis ever | 5391 | 73 | 2.2 | 1.5 |
| Once | 608 | 2 | 0.6 | 0.6 |
| 2–4 times | 1380 | 8 | 1.0 | 0.9 |
| 5–10 times | 806 | 9 | 1.9 | 1.4 |
| 11–50 times | 689 | 13 | 3.2 | 2.2 |
| >50 times | 731 | 28 | 6.7 | 3.1 |

* Adjusted odds ratio takes into account confounding factors: poor social integration, disturbed behavior, cigarette smoking, and place of upbringing.
Data from Zammit et al. (2002).

Although the existence of a causal relationship between cannabis use and long-term psychotic illness remains unproven, the increasing weight of evidence suggests that it is a possibility. But if cannabis use was an important cause of schizophrenia, one might expect to have seen an increase in the numbers of sufferers from this illness as cannabis use became more common in developed countries during the past 30 years, but there is no evidence that this occurred (Thornicroft, 1990; Degenhardt et al., 2003; Hickman et al., 2007). It is important to point out that the Swedish army study was the only one to use the diagnosis of schizophrenia as the outcome measure. All other cohort studies have simply looked for the presence or absence of some form of psychotic symptoms in adulthood. The syndrome is sometimes described as a schizophreniform psychosis, but it is not schizophrenia per se. With an odds ratio of 1.4, only a very small proportion of cannabis users (about 2%) might be expected to develop psychosis. The odds ratio of 15 linking cigarette smoking to lung cancer is far more alarming.

This is not to say that long-term cannabis use is harmless. Macleod et al. (2004) undertook a systematic review of 48 longitudinal cohort studies of cannabis and other drug users. Heavy long-term cannabis use was consistently associated with poor educational achievement, increased use of other psychoactive drugs, poor psychological health (including self-reported depression), and problematic behavior. Although the authors did not feel that there was enough evidence to attribute a causal link, the association of chronic cannabis use with poor psychosocial outcome remains.

It is also clear that cannabis can exacerbate the symptoms of existing psychotic illness. While schizophrenic patients like to use cannabis and other psychoactive drugs as a form of self-medication, cannabis can make the key symptoms of delusions and hallucinations worse, and it tends to counteract the antipsychotic effects of the drugs used to treat the illness (Negrete et al., 1986; Linzen et al., 1994; Castle and Murray, 2004). It would seem prudent to discourage the use of cannabis in patients with existing psychotic illness.

## Special Hazards of Smoked Marijuana

Traditionally the use of cannabis both in Oriental and Western medicine involved taking the drug by mouth, but most of the current recreational and medical use of the drug in the West involves the inhalation of marijuana smoke. Unfortunately, although smoking is a remarkably efficient means of delivering an accurately gauged dose of THC, it also carries with it special hazards. Although THC itself appears to be a relatively safe drug, the same cannot be said about marijuana smoke.

### Marijuana Smoke and Smoking Behavior

Although relatively little research has been done on the effects of marijuana smoke, a great deal is known about the toxic components in tobacco smoke and their biological effects. Marijuana smoke is very similar in chemical composition to tobacco smoke, so it is not unreasonable to suggest that our knowledge of the dangers of tobacco can provide useful predictions about the hazards of smoked marijuana. A burning tobacco cigarette has been described as a "miniature chemical factory." In addition to the large number of chemical components present in the dried plant material, hundreds of additional chemicals are created during the process of combustion. More than 6,000 chemical constituents have been identified in tobacco smoke and thousands more are present in trace amounts. The composition of tobacco smoke varies according to the manner in which the material is smoked. The nature of the wrapping paper, for example, alters the burning characteristics and consequently alters the chemical composition of the smoke. There is no reason to think that the same considerations do not also apply to marijuana. Table 6.2 summarizes the components present in smoke from a typical cigarette or marijuana joint. Apart from the fact that the former contains nicotine whereas the latter contains THC, the profiles are otherwise remarkably similar. Smoke consists of two components, the minute droplets present in the particulate phase and the various volatile chemicals or gases in the vapor phase. About 10% of the total weight of fresh tobacco or marijuana smoke is in the particulate phase, which contains most of the active drug (nicotine or THC). The particulate phase consists of minute droplets of condensed fluid, less than a quarter of a millionth of a micrometer in diameter (less than 1/1,000 of a millimeter), with as many as 5 billion droplets per milliliter of smoke. Both vapor and particulate phases of marijuana and tobacco smoke contain a number of toxic chemicals, several of which are known to be capable of promoting the development of cancers (carcinogens). Some reports have indicated that two of the most potent known carcinogens in tobacco smoke, benzanthracene and benzpyrene, are present in even higher amounts in marijuana smoke, although other measurements indicate that the amounts are similar in both types of smoke.

The manner in which experienced users smoke marijuana tends to enhance the potential dangers of taking the drug by this route. Marijuana smokers usually inhale more deeply than tobacco smokers and tend to hold their breath, in the belief that this increases the absorption of THC by the lungs. (In fact, the results of experimental studies in which both puff volume and breath hold duration were systematically varied show that while inhaling more deeply does increase the amount of THC absorbed, holding the breath for more than a few seconds has rather little effect. The concept seems to be based more on cultural myths than on reality.) The results of these differences in smoking behavior are quite

**Table 6.2.** Composition of Mainstream Smoke From Marijuana and Tobacco Cigarettes

|  | Marijuana Joint | Tobacco Cigarette |
|---|---|---|
| Average weight (mg) | 1,115.0 | 1,110.0 |
| Moisture (%) | 10.3 | 11.3 |
| **Gas Phase** | | |
| Carbon monoxide (mg) | 17.6 | 20.2 |
| Carbon dioxide (mg) | 57.3 | 65.0 |
| Ammonia (mg) | 0.3 | 0.2 |
| Hydrogen cyanide (μg) | 532.0 | 498.0 |
| Cyanogen (μg) | 19.0 | 20.0 |
| Isoprene (μg) | 83.0 | 310.0 |
| Acetaldehyde (μg) | 1,200.0 | 980.0 |
| Acetone (μg) | 443.0 | 578.0 |
| Acrolein (μg) | 92.0 | 85.0 |
| Acetonitrile (μg) | 132.0 | 123.0 |
| Benzene (μg) | 76.0 | 67.0 |
| Toluene (μg) | 112.0 | 108.0 |
| Vinyl chloride (ng)* | 5.4 | 12.4 |
| Dimethylnitrosamine (ng)* | 75.0 | 84.0 |
| Methylethylnitrosamine (ng)* | 27.0 | 30.0 |
| **Particulate Phase** | | |
| Total particulate matter (mg) | 22.7 | 39.0 |
| Phenol (μg) | 76.8 | 138.5 |
| o-Cresol (μg) | 17.9 | 24.0 |
| m- and p-Cresol (μg) | 54.4 | 65.0 |
| Dimethylphenol (μg) | 6.8 | 14.4 |
| Catechol (μg) | 188.0 | 328.0 |
| Cannabidiol (μg) | 190.0 | — |
| delta-9-THC (μg) | 820.0 | — |
| Cannabinol (μg) | 400.0 | — |
| Nicotine (μg) | — | 2,850.0 |
| N-nitrosonornicotine (ng)* | — | 390.0 |
| Naphthalene (μg) | 3.0 | 1.2 |
| 1-methylnaphthalene (μg) | 3.6 | 1.4 |
| Benz(a)anthracene (ng)* | 75.0 | 43.0 |
| Benz(a)pyrene (ng)* | 31.0 | 21.1 |

* Indicates known carcinogens.
Data from British Medical Association (1997).

Table 6.3. Comparison of Smoking Marijuana vs. Tobacco
Cigarette

|                              | Tobacco      | Marijuana    |
| ---------------------------- | ------------ | ------------ |
| Puff volume (mL)             | 49.4 ± 15.2  | 78.0 ± 22.8  |
| Puff duration (seconds)      | 2.4 ± 1.1    | 4.0 ± 2.2    |
| No. of puffs                 | 13.5 ± 4.0   | 8.5 ± 3.1    |
| Interval between puffs (sec) | 27.0 ± 8.2   | 37.6 ± 14.5  |
| Inhaled volume (liters)      | 1.31 ± 0.22  | 1.75 ± 0.52  |
| Smoke-retention time (sec)   | 3.5 ± 1.3    | 14.7 ± 10.2  |
| Inhaled particulates (O.D.)  | 4.9 ± 2.0    | 16.3 ± 6.3   |
| Particulates deposited (%)   | 64.0 ± 8.9   | 86.1 ± 6.71  |

Data are averages with 95% confidence limits obtained from 15 volunteers. Inhaled
particulates were assessed by optical density (O.D) measurements.
From Wu et al. (1988).


profound. Wu et al. (1988) compared the amounts of particulate matter
(tar) and carbon monoxide absorbed in 15 volunteers who were regular
tobacco and marijuana smokers. Results were compared after smoking a
single filter-tipped tobacco cigarette or a marijuana cigarette of comparable size. As compared with smoking tobacco, smoking marijuana resulted
in a fivefold greater absorption of carbon monoxide and four to five times
more tar was retained in the lungs (Table 6.3).

It is possible that the use of higher potency marijuana may reduce unwanted tar deposition. When low-potency (1.3% THC) joints were compared with higher potency material (2.7% THC) in experienced marijuana
smokers, Heishman et al. (1989) reported that smokers adjusted their smoking behavior so that they used smaller puff and inhalation volumes and
shorter puff duration for the higher THC material. Similar findings were
reported by Matthias et al. (1997), who also found that there was significantly less tar deposition when smokers used the higher potency material.
These data were obtained using the relatively low THC marijuana available
for research purposes in the United States at that time. Nowadays marijuana
with two to three times higher potency is readily available, and if the earlier
results can be extrapolated its use may result in even smaller tar deposition than previously. The conclusion seems to be that habitual marijuana

smokers could reduce the health hazards of smoking by using marijuana with a high THC content. Other possibilities include the use of water pipes, filters, or vaporizers to reduce the tar content of marijuana smoke before it enters the lungs (see Chapter 2).

## Effects of Marijuana Smoke on the Lungs

Since tobacco smoking is known to be the most important cause of chronic obstructive lung disease and lung cancer, it is reasonable to be concerned about the adverse effects of marijuana smoke on the lungs. There have been a number of attempts to address this question by exposing laboratory animals to marijuana smoke. After such exposure on a daily basis for periods of up to 30 months, extensive damage has been observed in the lungs of rats, dogs, and monkeys, but it is very difficult to extrapolate these findings to man as it is difficult or impossible to imitate the human exposure to marijuana smoke in any animal model. The various studies that have been undertaken in human marijuana smokers seem far more relevant, although here the problem is confounded by the fact that many marijuana smokers consume the drug with tobacco, making it difficult to disentangle the effects of the two agents. Professor Donald Tashkin and his colleagues at the Department of Medicine at the University of California Los Angeles has been a leader of research in this field (for review see Tashkin, 2005). In 1987 Tashkin reported the results of the first large-scale study of 144 volunteers who were heavy smokers of marijuana only. He compared these with 135 people who smoked tobacco and marijuana, as well as 70 smokers of tobacco only and 97 nonsmokers. Approximately 20% of both tobacco smokers and marijuana smokers reported the symptoms of chronic bronchitis (chronic cough and phlegm production), even though the marijuana smokers consumed only three to four joints a day versus more than 20 cigarettes for the tobacco smokers. In this study no additive effects were seen in those who smoked both marijuana and tobacco, although additive effects have been reported in other studies of this type. Ten years later Tashkin described a follow-up study of the groups studied earlier. He found that lung function in the tobacco smokers had continued to worsen over the 10-year period, particularly in the small airways, making them more liable to develop chronic obstructive lung disease later in life. No such decline was observed, however, in the marijuana smokers, suggesting that they may be less likely to develop such diseases as emphysema because of their smoking. Similar conclusions were reached from a study of 268 heavy marijuana smokers in Australia. After smoking regularly for an average of 19 years, they had a lower prevalence of asthma or emphysema than the general population. At the Kaiser Permanente health care group in California, a careful comparison of 452 daily marijuana smokers who never smoked tobacco with 450 nonsmokers of either substance revealed that the marijuana smokers had only a small increased risk of outpatient visits for respiratory illness (relative risk = 1.19) (Polen et al., 1993).

Some of the volunteers from Tashkin's Los Angeles studies were subjected to a saline rinse of their lungs in order to sample the population of white blood cells present. White cells are the soldiers of the immune system; they are attracted to regions of tissue inflammation or damage and help to kill and remove infectious microbial invaders and to remove damaged or dead cells and tissue debris. The large white cells known as macrophages are particularly important scavengers, which engulf and kill invading bacteria and fungi and remove damaged tissue. Approximately two to three times more macrophages were collected from the lungs of tobacco or marijuana smokers versus nonsmokers, suggesting the presence of an inflammatory response. The macrophages from both tobacco and marijuana smokers also showed significant impairments in their ability to kill and engulf fungi (*Candida albicans*) or bacteria (*Staphylococcus aureus*). The macrophages from smokers were also less able to generate some of the chemical toxins (e.g., superoxide) that they normally use to kill invading micro-organisms, or the chemicals known as cytokines, which help to activate further inflammatory and immune system responses. In addition, the macrophages were impaired in their ability to attack and kill cancer cells (small cell cancers) in vitro. Studies in animals have confirmed these findings, showing that exposure of macrophages to marijuana smoke in vitro impairs their function, and that exposure of rats to marijuana smoke in vivo makes them less able to inactivate bacteria (*S. aureus*) delivered by aerosol to the lungs. The animal studies also indicated that the toxic effects of marijuana smoke on the immune defenses were not due to THC but to some other components of the marijuana smoke, since smoke from THC-extracted herbal material remained toxic. These findings suggest that like tobacco smokers, marijuana smokers are likely to be more susceptible to respiratory tract infections and possibly less able to defend against the development of lung cancers. An added complication is that some batches of herbal cannabis may be contaminated with fungi (e.g., *Aspergillus* species) that could themselves cause lung infections. This could be a particular hazard to AIDS patients whose immune defenses are already compromised.

A similar concern is the contamination of some U.S. supplies of herbal cannabis by the herbicide paraquat, used by the U.S. government to destroy cannabis crops in the United States and Mexico. Paraquat has potent toxic effects on the lung, causing inflammation and congestion that can be life threatening. Fortunately, this hazard seems less important now than it was a few years ago.

## Marijuana Smoking and Lung Cancer

THC does not appear to be carcinogenic, but there is plenty of evidence that the tar derived from marijuana smoke is. Bacteria exposed to marijuana tar develop mutations in the standard Ames test for carcinogenicity and hamster lung cells in tissue culture develop accelerated malignant transformations within 3 to 6 months of exposure to tobacco or marijuana smoke. Painting marijuana tar on the skin of mice also leads to premalignant lesions. But is there any evidence that this happens in the lungs of marijuana smokers?

As part of Tashkin's original 1987 study, some of the volunteers were examined in more detail for evidence of damage to the airways. Visual examination of the large airways with a bronchoscope showed evidence of increased redness and swelling and increased mucus production in a large proportion of both marijuana and tobacco smokers relative to nonsmokers. Excision of minute amounts of tissue (biopsies) from the lining of the airways allowed microscopic examination. This revealed abnormal cell changes in both marijuana and tobacco smokers. These included an abnormal proliferation of mucus-producing cells and a reduced number of ciliated cells (these are normally present in the lining of the airways; the movement of their hair-like cilia helps to clear the lungs of mucus and debris). These changes could explain the chronic cough and overproduction of phlegm reported by tobacco and marijuana smokers. A more sinister observation was the presence of abnormal cells resembling those normally seen in skin (squamous metaplasia) in the lungs of smokers. These changes are thought to represent premalignant precursors for the development of lung cancer. The possible premalignant cells were seen to an even greater extent in the lungs of volunteers who smoked both marijuana and tobacco. Similar findings of premalignant changes in the lungs of cannabis smokers have been confirmed in other laboratories (reviewed by Mehra et al., 2006) and extended by examining lung biopsies from marijuana and tobacco smokers to see if the cells express certain genes that must be activated for normal lung cells to transform into cancer cells with some positive results (Tashkin, 2005; Mehra et al., 2006). The changes observed are worrying as they may indicate that series of precancerous changes take place in the lungs of marijuana smokers, similar to those which occur in tobacco smokers, the end result of which might be to significantly increase the likelihood of developing lung cancer.

The discovery of the link between cigarette smoking and lung cancer was one of the great achievements of medical research in this century. The initial reports in 1950 from Britain and the United States were based on two very large case-control studies. Subsequently, a great deal more has been learned from follow-up studies in large groups of smokers and nonsmokers. One such study involved asking all the doctors in Britain about their smoking habits. More than 40,000 doctors agreed to take part in a long-term study to see what effect their smoking habits might have on their health. The study started in 1951, and Doll et al. (2005), in one of his last publications, described the results of a 50-year follow-up of this group. The results were alarming; not only was the risk of dying from lung cancer increased in the cigarette smokers, but also so were the risks of dying from 23 other causes, including cancers of the mouth, throat, larynx, pancreas, and bladder and such obstructive lung diseases as asthma and emphysema. The authors concluded that they had previously substantially underestimated the hazards of the long-term use of tobacco. The long-term follow-up data showed that about half of all regular cigarette smokers will eventually be killed by their habit.

It is hard to overestimate the importance of tobacco smoking as the principal avoidable cause of death in the modern world. More people die from smoking tobacco than any other single cause. Worldwide, some 3 million deaths a year can be attributed to tobacco, and this is likely to rise to 10 million a year in 30 to 40 years' time (Peto et al., 1996). In developed countries tobacco is responsible for nearly 25% of all male deaths and 17% of women. People in the developing countries started smoking later in the twentieth century, but they are catching up fast in the tobacco mortality statistics. The results of a recent study in China, involving an analysis of more than 1 million deaths, make some frightening predictions. Cigarette smoking in China has increased dramatically in the recent past—almost quadrupling since 1980. About two thirds of men over the age of 25 smoke, and about half of these will die prematurely because of their tobacco habit. This implies that eventually 100 million of the 300 million young men now alive and aged 0 to 29 will be killed by tobacco (half dying in middle age, half in old age) (Liu et al., 1998).

But is there any evidence for an increased risk of cancer in cannabis smokers? One of the few large-scale studies of the health consequences of marijuana smoking was reported by Sidney et al. (1997). The authors studied a cohort of 65,171 men and women undergoing health checks at the Kaiser Permanente health care organization in California between 1979 and 1985. The health of these subjects was then followed for an average of a further 10 years. A total of nearly 27,000 people admitted to being either current or former marijuana users (defined as ever having smoked more than six times). Over the period of the study 182 tobacco-related cancers were detected, of which 97 were lung malignancies. No effects of former or current marijuana use on the risk of any cancers were found. However, although this study involved large numbers, almost all the marijuana smokers were young (15 to 39) and the follow-up period was relatively short. Such a study could not have been expected to detect any relationship between marijuana and lung cancer if the lag period were comparable to that seen with tobacco. More recent systematic surveys of the published literature have concluded that there is no evidence for a link between cannabis and lung cancer, or a variety of other cancers for which an association has sometimes been claimed (e.g., cancer of the head or neck, oral cancer) (Hashibe et al., 2005; Mehra et al., 2006). In a follow-up study Hashibe et al. (2006) compared the drug history of 1,212 patients with cancer of the lungs or upper airways/digestive tract with 1,041 cancer-free controls. After allowing for the known effects of cigarette smoking, they found no increased risk of any of these cancers (lung, oral, pharyngeal, or esophageal) in cannabis smokers. Indeed, for lung cancer there was even a reduced risk ratio for cannabis smokers versus controls (odds ratio = 0.62), despite the fact that some subjects had smoked cannabis once a day for more than 30 years. The authors concluded:

> Our results suggest that the association of these cancers with marijuana, even, long term or heavy use, is not strong and may be below practically detectable limits.

But one of the reasons why we should continue to be seriously concerned about the possible link between marijuana smoking and lung cancer is that it could take a very long time for such a relationship to become manifest. Cigarette smoking became common among men in the developed world during the first decades of this century, but it was not until 30 to 40 years later that the first evidence of a link between tobacco smoking and lung cancer was obtained. Even though cigarette consumption has declined significantly in many developed countries, deaths from tobacco-related diseases will continue to rise for many years to come, particularly among women, for whom cigarette smoking was not common until the 1930s or 1940s. Such long lag periods between cause and effect are hard to comprehend. The relationship between cigarette smoking and lung cancer is very complex. The increased risk of developing lung cancer depends far more strongly on the duration of cigarette smoking than on the number of cigarettes consumed each day. Thus, while smoking three times as many cigarettes a day does increase the lung cancer risk approximately threefold, smoking for 30 years as opposed to smoking for 15 years does not simply double the lung cancer risk, it increases the risk by 20-fold, and smoking for 45 years as opposed to 15 years increases the lung cancer risk 100-fold (Peto, 1986).

The reasons underlying the relationship between the duration of tobacco smoking and the development of lung cancer are unknown, but they might apply to marijuana smokers as well. To argue that because a link has not yet been established between marijuana smoking and lung cancer no such link is likely to exist is unwarranted. Since the widespread use of marijuana as a recreational drug is a fairly recent development in the Western world, large numbers of people have not yet been exposed to marijuana smoking for long enough for any link to become clear. The following comments on tobacco smoking could well apply also to marijuana:

Among regular cigarette smokers, the excess lung cancer risk depends strongly not only on smoking habits during the past few years, but also on smoking habits during early adult life. Hence, current lung cancer rates in countries where smoking among young adults became widespread less than half a century ago may be serious underestimates of the eventual magnitude of the tobacco-induced lung cancer hazard. (Peto, 1986)

## Summary

1. The safety profile of the active ingredient of cannabis, THC, is good. It has very low toxicity both in the short and in the longer term. Some of the acute effects of the drug, however, including the liability to cause unpleasant psychotic reactions in some and intoxication in others and to cause temporary impairments in skilled motor and cognitive functions, limit the usefulness of THC as a medicine. There appears to be only a narrow window between the desired and the undesired effects.

2. Because of the cardiovascular effects of THC and its propensity to make schizophrenic symptoms worse, patients with cardiovascular disease or schizophrenia are not suitable subjects for cannabis-based medicines. As with most other CNS drugs, cannabis use should be avoided during pregnancy.

3. The safety of smoked marijuana is questionable. It causes chronic bronchitis in a substantial proportion of regular users, and the potential risk that in the longer term an association may be found with cancers of the respiratory tract makes it unsafe to recommend for any long-term use.

4. The possible link between teenage use of cannabis and the subsequent development of psychotic illness means that every effort should be made to educate young people about the potential dangers of cannabis use. But this is unlikely to represent a significant deterrent to the medical use of cannabis in adult patients.

The Institute of Medicine (1999) in their report *Marijuana and Medicine* summarized the safety issues succinctly:

Marijuana is not a completely benign substance. It is a powerful drug with a variety of effects. However, except for the harms associated with smoking, the adverse effects of marijuana use are within the range of effects tolerated for other medications.

The Police Foundation review in 2000 also concluded:

By any of the major criteria of harm—mortality, morbidity, toxicity, addictiveness and relationship with crime—cannabis is less harmful than any of the other major illicit drugs, or than alcohol or tobacco.

# 7

## The Recreational Use
## of Cannabis

The use of cannabis as a recreational drug was almost unknown in the West until the 1950s and only became widespread during the 1960s. The exposure of large numbers of young American soldiers to cannabis during the Vietnam War was an important contributory factor (see, for example, the famous Vietnam War movies *Platoon* and *The Deer Hunter*). As Napoleon's army brought cannabis to Europe from their Egyptian campaign, the returning GIs brought cannabis to the United States. The use of cannabis by young people on both sides of the Atlantic was closely linked to the protest and rebellion experienced by the 1960s generation:

> The most profound example of the ability of marijuana to raise mass social consciousness occurred during the Vietnam War era, on both the home front and the battle front. The spread of marijuana use to almost an entire generation of middle-class youth who came of age in the 1960's is inextricable from the dramatic changes in social, political, spiritual and cultural values that mark that era. Cannabis did not kidnap them or their collective consciousness: the generation was ready for marijuana. (Robinson, 1996)

According to popular mythology, cannabis really started to enter the mass consciousness sometime in 1964 when the Beatles met Bob Dylan at an airport in America. He offered them a joint in the VIP lounge. Only Ringo tried it then, but soon they were all enthusiastic users and role models.

By the beginning of the new millennium another generation had replaced the rebellious youth of 40 years ago, a new generation far less extravagant in their lifestyle, more serious, and no longer feeling the deep sense of alienation from traditional society that many young people experienced in the 1960s. To this generation cannabis is a part of their culture, no longer a gesture of rebellion. Many of the parents and even the grandparents of today's generation of cannabis users themselves belonged to the 1960s and 1970s group of marijuana smokers.

Cannabis has become by far the most widely used illicit drug in the Western world. It ranks as the third most commonly used recreational drug after alcohol and tobacco. Whereas detailed information is available on the consumption of alcohol and tobacco, the health problems they cause, and the consequent economic costs to society, such information is lacking in such precise detail for cannabis. The use of cannabis occurs in an underground world of illegality. In most countries, according to a United Nations Convention (see Chapter 8), cannabis is considered as a Schedule 1 drug (i.e., a dangerous narcotic with no accepted medical usefulness). Possession of cannabis, cultivation of the cannabis plant, and trafficking are criminal offenses, some of which can carry severe penalties. It is not surprising that the users and suppliers of this illicit drug are not always willing to provide detailed information about it, but nevertheless, millions of people are regular users.

## Prevalence

For the reasons previously mentioned it is difficult to obtain accurate figures on the prevalence of cannabis use, but there are some useful sources. In the United States the National Survey on Drug Use and Health has produced a valuable annual report since 1972 (http://www.oas.samhsa.gov), and data are also available from the National Institute on Drug Abuse through their Monitoring the Future Study (http://www.drugabuse.gov/infofacts/ marijuana.html); in the United Kingdom the British Crime Survey includes data on drug use (http://www.homeoffice.gov.uk/rds/bcs1.html). The European Monitoring Centre for Drugs and Drug Abuse provides annual data from 29 European countries (http://stats06.emcdda.europa.eu). As many as one third of the entire population aged 15 to 50 in many Western countries admit to having used cannabis at least once. Consumption is highest in the younger age groups. In the United States more than half of 18- to 25-year-olds have tried cannabis (National Survey on Drug Use and Health, 2005; http://www.oas.samsha.gov); in most European countries the proportion of this age group who have used cannabis is lower, with the range being 20% to 40%. Table 7.1 summarizes patterns of cannabis use in different European countries, using data from the latest available surveys; regular cannabis use is generally considerably lower than in the United States (less than half in most countries), with young people in Britain and Spain standing out as the most frequent consumers.

**Table 7.1.** European 15- to 34-Year-Olds Who Used Cannabis in the Past Month

| Country | Percentage | Country | Percentage |
| --- | --- | --- | --- |
| Belgium | 5.9 | Italy | 8.6 |
| Czech Republic | 9.8 | Hungary | 2.8 |
| Denmark | 5.6 | Netherlands | 7.0 |
| Germany | 7.6 | Austria | 6.4 |
| Greece | 1.5 | Poland | 2.7 |
| Ireland | 4.3 | United Kingdom | 11.6 |
| Norway | 4.5 | Spain | 13.4 |

From the European Monitoring Centre for Drugs and Drug Abuse 2006 Report. Available at: http://stats06.emcdda.europa.eu/en/elements/gpstab16-en.html.

Patterns of consumption over the years have varied differently in various countries. In the United States, statistics provided by the National Institute on Drug Abuse through their Monitoring the Future Study give a detailed picture of cannabis use among teenagers. Cannabis became very popular among young people in the United States during the 1970s, reaching a peak in 1979, when more than 60% of 12th-grade students in American high schools (average age 18) admitted ever having used the drug, and 10% reported that they were daily users. There was then a marked drop in consumption during the 1980s as health fears grew. Consumption, however, increased again during the 1990s and now appears to have stabilized or to have declined somewhat in recent years (Bell et al., 1997) (Table 7.2).

Patterns of consumption in most European countries have lagged behind those in the United States, but most countries did not experience the substantial drop in consumption seen in the United States during the 1980s. In Britain, government statistics indicate that there has been a significant decline in cannabis use by young people (16- to 24-year-olds) in the period 2000–2006 (Table 7.3). Despite this, almost one in three of 16- to 24-year-old men almost one in five of 16- to 24-year-old women report using cannabis some time in the past year.

The great majority of people who try cannabis do so experimentally. Unlike tobacco, where a high proportion of first-time users go on to become lifetime smokers, most cannabis users do not become regular users of the

Table 7.2. Percentage of 12th Graders in the
United States (About 18 Years Old) Who
Have Used Cannabis

| Year | In Past Year | In Past Month |
|------|--------------|---------------|
| 1994 | 30.7 | 19.0 |
| 1995 | 34.7 | 21.2 |
| 1996 | 35.8 | 21.9 |
| 1997 | 38.5 | 23.7 |
| 1998 | 37.5 | 22.8 |
| 1999 | 37.8 | 23.1 |
| 2000 | 36.5 | 21.6 |
| 2001 | 37.0 | 22.4 |
| 2002 | 36.2 | 21.5 |
| 2003 | 34.9 | 21.2 |
| 2004 | 34.3 | 19.8 |
| 2005 | 33.6 | 19.8 |

Data from the National Institute on Drug Abuse (2005); (http://
www.drugabuse.gov/infofacts/marijuana.html)


Table 7.3. Percentage of 16- to 24-Year-Olds in
Britain Who Have Used Cannabis

| Year | In Past Year | In Past Month |
|------|--------------|---------------|
| 1996 | 26.0 | 16.1 |
| 1998 | 28.2 | 18.0 |
| 2000 | 27.0 | 17.4 |
| 2001–2002 | 26.9 | 17.1 |
| 2002–2003 | 25.8 | 16.2 |
| 2003–2004 | 24.8 | 15.6 |
| 2004–2005* | 23.5 | 14.1 |
| 2005–2006 | 21.5** | 13.0** |

* Cannabis downgraded from Category B to C in January 2004.
** Decline in use between 2000 and 2005–2006 is statistically significant.
Data from British Crime Survey; (http://www.homeoffice.gov.uk/rds/bcs1.
html)

drug. There is no agreed-upon definition of a regular user; it could mean anything from someone who took the drug a few times a year on special occasions to someone consuming the drug several times a day. National Institute on Drug Abuse data on American 18-year-olds in 2005 show that nearly one in five admitted to having used cannabis at least once during the past month and 5% reported that they were daily users. A World Health Organization (WHO) survey in 1997 reported that in Canada a quarter of children aged 15 to 17 were current users (WHO, 1997); in Australia as many as 15% of adult men and 7% of women were weekly users; and in most European countries around 5% of the adult population were current users. In Britain, data from the British Crime Survey 2005/06 (cf Table 7.3) for the adult population (aged 16 to 59) indicated that 5% had consumed cannabis during the past month, and as with 16- to 24-year-olds there had been a significant decline in use since 2000. It seems likely that only relatively small numbers of people on either side of the Atlantic use cannabis once a week or more, but if the definition of regular user includes those who use cannabis only a few times each month, then there are estimated to be more than 3 million cannabis users in Britain. The definition of regular user, however, encompasses a wide range of consumption patterns.

## How Is Cannabis Consumed and Where Does It Come From?

In the United States the most common form of the drug is herbal marijuana or sensemilla (dried female flowering heads), nowadays frequently cultivated indoors and usually smoked with tobacco but also quite frequently on its own. The majority of users prepare their own hand-rolled joints, or *blunts*, which are cigars emptied of their tobacco content and filled with marijuana.

The great majority of the supplies of this material during the 1970s were from cannabis plants grown on farms in the southern United States and in northern Mexico. The U.S. government's campaigns to eliminate these supplies (often by spraying the cannabis fields with the herbicide paraquat) led to imports from further afield. Colombia and certain Caribbean countries, notably Jamaica, became more important. In recent years there has been a large increase in the consumption of home-grown cannabis—often using modern strains of plant yielding a high tetrahydrocannabinol (THC) content and grown secretly indoors with artificial lighting. This has become a growth industry, particularly in the Western states of the United States and in British Columbia in Canada. The Internet provides a rich source of advice on how to grow cannabis indoors, detailing the optimum heating and lighting needed and where to obtain the necessary seeds and equipment. For a modest investment small growers can obtain the equipment for a modest-sized indoor growing room; several crops can be harvested each year and they can expect to make more than US $100,000 a year of tax-free income.

In the quiet countryside just outside Vancouver B.C., an ambitious young entrepreneur surveys a blindingly bright room filled with lovely plants—dozens of stalks of high-power marijuana. Almost ready for harvest, they hold thread-like, resin-frosted pot flowers, rust and white "buds" thickening in a base of green-and-purple leaves. The room reeks of citrus and menthol, a drug-rich musk lingering on fingertips and clothes.

"There's no way I won't make a million dollars." Says the entrepreneur, David. He runs several other sites like this one, reaping upwards of $80,000 in a ten–twelve week growing cycle. Says he: "Even if they bust for one, I'm covered." (http://www.reggaerunnins.com/cash_crop_110603.htm)

This is typical of the thousands of small high-tech marijuana grows—as the indoor farms are known in Canada. Marijuana growing has become a big business in Canada and is likely to get bigger because of the cannabis-tolerant atmosphere. Canadians seem loath to stamp out what has emerged as their most valuable agricultural product—bigger than wheat, cattle, or timber and estimated to earn $5 to $10 billion (in US dollars) annually (http://www.reaggaerunniins.com/cash_crop_110603.htm).

A recent report estimated that marijuana had also become the largest cash crop in the United States, exceeding $35 billion annually, far more than such traditional heartland staples as corn, soybeans, and hay (Gettman, 2006). California is responsible for more than a third of the cannabis harvest, with an estimated production of $13.8 billion, exceeding the value of the state's fruit and vegetable production (Table 7.4)

**Table 7.4.** Total U.S. Marijuana
Cultivation in 2006

| State | Pounds Produced | Total Value |
|---|---|---|
| California | 8.6 million | $13.8 billion |
| Tennessee | 3 million | $4.8 billion |
| Kentucky | 2.8 million | $4.5 billion |
| Hawaii | 2.4 million | $3.8 million |
| Washington | 641,354 | $1 billion |

From Gettman (2006).

The Independent Drug Monitoring Unit (IDMU) has provided some
of the most detailed information available on the recreational use of cannabis in Britain. A number of surveys of cannabis users were carried out
between 1982 and 2005, including those who attended outdoor pop music
festivals. The results of these surveys, involving thousands of users, are available on their Web site (http://www.idmu.co.uk/canuse05.htm). In Britain, as
in the United States, virtually all recreational use (96%) is by smoking,
although in Britain this is nearly always with tobacco. The most common
form of the drug in Britain until recently was imported resin. The cheapest
is from Morocco (*soap bar*), often heavily adulterated and contaminated.
Better quality resin from Lebanon and Nepal is also available. A relative
newcomer is *polm*, produced by compression of high-quality, finely sieved
resin bracts; the price can be as high as £200 per ounce. But resin has now
been overtaken by *skunk*—the generic name now given in Britain to cannabis grown indoors under controlled conditions.

Cannabis is most commonly smoked with tobacco in hand-rolled joints
or *spliffs*, although some herbal cannabis is smoked without tobacco, and resin
may also be smoked in pipes or bongs. In addition, less common forms of consumption are also used by some. These include *hot knives*, in which a piece
of cannabis resin is held between two heated blades and the resulting smoke
inhaled, and the *bucket* technique, in which the smoke from a smoldering
piece of cannabis resin is captured in a bottle or bucket and then inhaled. A
small proportion of users take the drug in food or drink, although as many as
a quarter of the IDMU group reported that they did this occasionally.

Most cannabis resin in the United Kingdom is imported from Morocco or other parts of North Africa, with smaller amounts from Pakistan, Afghanistan, Lebanon, and the Netherlands. Skunk is home grown or imported from the Netherlands (*nederwiet*). As in Canada and the United States, there has been a rapid increase in illegal cannabis farms in Britain. The costs of resin or herbal cannabis in 2004 ranged from less than £10 per one-eighth ounce (3.5 g) for Moroccan "soap" to more than £20 per one-eighth ounce for skunk—prices had fallen to less than half what they were 10 years earlier. The imported resin is often adulterated with other materials, commonly with caryophyllene, an aromatic constituent of cloves. Poor-quality skunk may be contaminated with flour or even with powdered glass to give it the appearance of high-quality powdery and glistening female flower heads. In most European countries prices are similar, in the range 5 to 10 Eu/gram.

## Patterns of Recreational Use

The IDMU surveys of regular cannabis users in Britain have revealed a wide range of differing patterns of use. More than half of this self-reported group admitted to being daily users. In 2004 the average monthly consumption of cannabis by daily users amounted to 56 g (about 20 ounces), equivalent to six to seven joints per day. Less frequent regular users consumed much less, 5 to 15 g per month. Among those admitting use more than once a day, average consumption was 66 g of resin per month. The maximum levels of consumption reported were 150 to 200 g/month. This wide range of consumption levels is illustrated in Figures 7.1 and 7.2. A majority of users consume less than 15 g of resin per month and many do not take the drug on a daily basis. The wide range of cannabis consumption resembles that of alcohol, which is also consumed over a wide range of intakes, whereas a large majority of cigarette smokers fall within a narrow range of 15 to 40 cigarettes a day.

The IDMU data confirmed a downward trend in cannabis use among drug users as a whole. In 1994, among 1,333 young people who admitted to using any illegal drug, 87% were regular or daily cannabis users, but a survey of 2,959 drug users 10 years later in 2004 revealed only 36% as regular

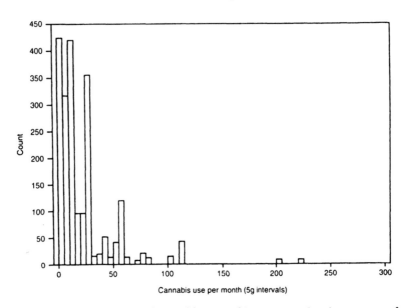

Figure 7.1. Distribution of monthly cannabis consumption in a group of 2469 regular cannabis users in Britain, surveyed between 1994 and 1997 by the Independent Drug Monitoring Unit. (Data provided to the House of Lords, Select Committee on Science and Technology, 1998.)

or daily cannabis users. This presumably reflects the increased popularity of other psychoactive drugs, notably cocaine and ecstasy.

Neil Montgomery, a social anthropologist from Edinburgh, Scotland, gave evidence to the House of Lords (1998). He divided recreational cannabis users in the United Kingdom into three categories:

- *Casual*: Irregular use, in amount of up to 1 g resin at a time to an annual total of no more than 28 g (1 ounce)
- *Regular*: Regular use, typically three to four smokes of a joint or pipe a day, equivalent to about 14 g cannabis resin (half-ounce) per month

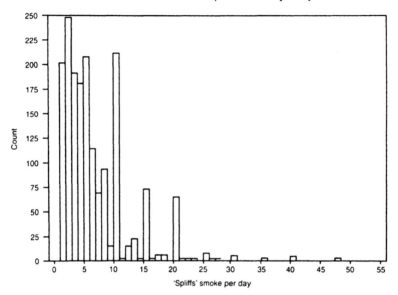

**Distribution of number of 'spliffs' smoked per day**

'Spliffs' smoke per day

**Figure 7.2.** Distribution of number of marijuana cigarettes (*spliffs*) smoked per day in 2469 regular cannabis users in Britain, surveyed between 1994 and 1997 by the Independent Drug Monitoring Unit. (Data provided to the House of Lords, Select Committee on Science and Technology, 1998.)

• *Heavy*: Only about 5% of total users, but they are more or less permanently stoned, using more than 3.5 g resin per day and 28 g (1 ounce) or more each week

His figures, based on his own research with more than 200 cannabis users, are consistent with those provided by the IDMU. Montgomery pointed out:

The extent to which a heavy user can consume cannabis is largely unappreciated....These are people who have become dependent on cannabis; they are psychologically addicted to the almost constant consumption of cannabis....Becoming stoned and remaining stoned throughout the day is their prime directive.

The maximum consumption figures reported by Montgomery and by IDMU correspond to large intakes of THC. People consuming more than 5 g cannabis resin a day may have a daily intake of as much as 200 to 300 mg THC. These are by no means the highest figures reported in the literature, however. There are reliable records of people in the Caribbean consuming as much as 50 g cannabis per day. One study of cannabis users in Greece estimated an average daily intake of 7.5 g (quarter ounce) a day. It is likely that such heavy users have become tolerant to most of the effects of THC. Montgomery estimated that the heavy users might need as much as eight times more cannabis than more modest consumers to become high.

The IDMU surveys refer mainly to young cannabis users, and illicit use continues to be far more common among those under the age of 30. Nearly all surveys also show that recreational cannabis use is about twice as common in men as in women. The IDMU noted, however, that although prevalence decreased in those over the age of 30, this may reflect more a cultural divide between generations and this situation may not hold in the future. They note that the British Crime Survey 1991–1996 reported the greatest proportional increases in cannabis exposure in older age groups. Lifetime prevalence more than doubled between 1991 and 1996 in those aged 40 to 44 (from 15% to 30%) and trebled in the 45 to 59 age group (from 3% to 10%). In the United States the statistics also showed a significant increase in illicit drug use (mainly marijuana) between 2000 and 2004 by those aged 55 to 59 years. This may reflect the entry of the more drug-experienced baby boomer generation into this age group.

## What Are the Effects of Recreational Cannabis Use?

Harrison Pope and colleagues conducted anonymous questionnaire studies of illicit drug use at the same academic institution in the United States on four occasions over a 20-year period (1969, 1978, 1989, 1999), each time obtaining data from several hundred students (Pope et al., 2001b). Their results provide a valuable picture of marijuana use on the American campus over this period. The incidence of marijuana use fluctuated widely, with weekly use reaching a peak of 26% of respondents in 1978 but falling to 5.7% in 1989. Marijuana was by far the most commonly used drug, followed by alcohol. There were no differences between drug-using versus non–drug-using students in most indices assessed; these included academic performance as measured by grade-point averages, or participation in college athletic, social, and political activities. Whereas drug users in the 1969 survey reported a significantly higher level of "alienation from American society," this was no longer true 20 years later. By then there were only two factors that distinguished drug users from nonusers: they tended to visit a psychiatrist more often (although this did not seem to be directly attributable to drug use) and had more heterosexual experience (86% of the 1989 drug-user group reported having had intercourse with at least one partner, whereas only 52% of nonusers reported this). A follow-up study 10 years later in 1999 at the same college showed cannabis use to have remained stable but use of other illicit drugs had decreased, except for ecstasy, whose use increased markedly after 1990 (Pope et al., 2001b).

Kandel et al. (1996) surveyed 7,611 students, aged 13 to 18, in 53 New York State schools. Of these, 995 had experience of marijuana, but there was no evidence that this had any significant impact on their school performance or their family relationships, whereas the small number (121) of crack cocaine users showed significant impairments in both.

In terms of adverse effects, Berke and Hernton (1977) in their survey of 522 British cannabis users found that about half of the group reported feeling physically ill on one or more occasions after taking cannabis, the most frequent symptoms being nausea, sickness, and vomiting. These symptoms occurred shortly after taking the drug and were transient (15 to 30 minutes). Dizziness, headache, or exhaustion was the next most frequent physical symptom. A quarter of the group reported that on occasion they had unpleasant mental experiences. The most common symptoms were paranoia, fear, depression, anxiety, derealization, or hallucinations. A small number of people (49 of 522) admitted committing a socially irresponsible act while under the influence of the drug, the most common being driving while stoned, fighting, or inappropriate sexual activity (although only 1% cited "better sex" as one of the effects of the drug).

In assessing what effect cannabis has on recreational users, the IDMU survey data on British users are again a valuable source of information.

Table 7.5. Most Common Positive Benefits
Reported by 2794 British Cannabis Users

| Effect | % Reporting |
| --- | --- |
| Relaxation/relief from stress | 25.6 |
| Insight/personal development | 8.7 |
| Antidepressant/happy | 4.9 |
| Cognitive benefit | 2.9 |
| Creativity | 2.3 |
| Sociability | 2.0 |
| **Health Effects** | |
| Pain relief | 6.1 |
| Respiratory benefit | 2.4 |
| Improved sleep | 1.6 |
| Total reporting positive effects | 57.8 |

While the majority of publications on this topic stress the adverse effects of cannabis, the overwhelming message from the British users was positive. When asked to rate their attitudes to a variety of psychoactive drugs, cannabis was given the highest positive rating, followed by ecstasy and lysergic acid diethylamide (LSD). Negative attitude ratings were given to solvents, cocaine, heroin, and tranquilizers. Table 7.5 summarizes the positive benefits claimed by the regular cannabis users. The most common were relaxation, a sense of calm, and relief from stress. A variety of medical benefits were also reported, although only 2.8% of the group reported that medical use was their principle reason for taking the drug.

When asked why they took cannabis, more than 50% cited relaxation, pleasure, recreation, or social reasons. While the majority enjoyed the drug-induced experience, 21% of the group reported having experienced adverse effects on some occasion. These are summarized in Table 7.6. Adverse psychological effects (apathy, paranoia, anxiety, and panic) were the most common. Very few users admitted to being dependent on cannabis.

Users were also asked whether they had ever been involved in road traffic accidents, and the results indicated that accident rates among this group of young people were not significantly different from the national for all drivers in this age group. The conclusion that cannabis does not appear

Table 7.6. Adverse Effects Attributed
to Cannabis Experienced "Regularly"
by British Users in 1999 Independent
Drug Monitoring Unit Survey

| Effect | % Reporting |
| --- | --- |
| Apathy | 20.9 |
| Balance | 8.3 |
| Paranoia | 6.4 |
| Impaired memory | 3.9 |
| Anxiety/panic | 3.8 |
| Chest problems | 3.5 |
| Withdrawal | 1.5 |
| Total reporting problems | 21.0 |

to be a major cause of road accidents is, however, regarded as tentative
pending further data.

## The Potency of Illicit Marijuana

One of the claims frequently made by opponents of the recreational use
of marijuana is that cannabis today is far more potent than the relatively
harmless low-THC herbal material smoked by the flower-power generation
of the 1960s and 1970s (see also Chapter 1). It is claimed that the supplies
of cannabis available today are 10, 20, or even 40 times more potent than
previously. These fears have been fueled by the oft-quoted statement made
by the U.S. drug czar John Walters in 2002:

> Parents are often unaware that today's marijuana is different from that of a
> generation ago, with potency levels 10 to 20 times stronger than the mari-
> juana with which they were familiar. (Washington Post, May 1, 2002)

As Professor Heather Ashton put it in her evidence to the House of
Lords (1998) enquiry:

> The increase in potency is important because the physical and psychologi-
> cal effects of cannabinoids (THC and others) are dose-related: the bigger

the dose the greater the effect. Most of the research on cannabis was carried out in the 1970s using relatively small doses, and much of that research is obsolete today. The acute and long term effects of the present high dose use of cannabis have not been systematically studied.

But is it really true that commonly available cannabis today is so much more potent? And does it matter? For more than 20 years the U.S. government has sponsored the Potency Monitoring Project at the University of Mississippi that has been measuring the THC content of thousands of seized samples submitted by law enforcement agencies throughout the United States. There has been considerable fluctuation from year to year in the data—but it is clear that if there has been any progressive increase in the potency of herbal marijuana, it represents not much more than a doubling in THC content over more than 20 years (King et al., 2004). The European Monitoring Centre for Drugs and Drug Abuse undertook a survey of cannabis potencies in several European countries (King et al., 2004). There were considerable variations from year to year, but there were no detectable upward trends in the potency of imported cannabis resin (average 5% to 10% THC). On the other hand, the potency of cultivated cannabis (*skunk* or the Dutch version *nederwiet*) had shown significant increases in the past 20 years, and this was particularly marked in the Netherlands, where cultivation methods were most advanced. Pijlman et al. (2005) carried out an analysis of the potency of various varieties of cannabis available in Dutch coffee shops and found significant increases in potency in locally grown herbal material (*nederwiet*) or resin (*nederhasj*) each year in the period 2000–2004, while the potency of imported cannabis remained fairly constant (Table 7.7).

In Britain, the U.K. Government Forensic Science Service provided data to the House of Lords (1998) enquiry on the THC content of cannabis samples seized in the United Kingdom. They made the following statements:

Cannabis resin, a wholly imported material, has a mean THC content of 4–5 per cent, although the range is from less than 1% to around 10%. This pattern has remained unchanged for many years.

Until about eight years ago, "home grown" cannabis was a poor quality product often grown in greenhouses or on windowsills and normally for

Table 7.7. Percentage THC Content of Cannabis Products in the
Netherlands

| Product | 2000 | 2001 | 2002 | 2003 | 2004 |
|---|---|---|---|---|---|
| Nederwiet | 8.6 | 11.3 | 15.1 | 18.1 | 20.4* |
| Nederhasj | 20.7 | 15.7 | 33.0 | 35.8 | 39.3* |
| Imported herbal | 5.0 | 5.3 | 6.6 | 6.2 | 7.0 |
| Imported resin | 11.0 | 12.1 | 17.5 | 16.6 | 18.2* |

* Statistically significantly different from 2000 to 2001.
Data from Pijlman et al. (2005).

personal use. However, the introduction of a number of horticultural techniques has lead to the widespread and large scale domestic indoor cultivation
of cannabis with a much higher THC content. These techniques include
hydroponics, artificial lighting, control of "day" length, heating and ventila-
tion, cloning of "mother plants," and perhaps most importantly, the development of plant varieties which produce higher THC levels. The mean
THC content of so-called hydroponic cannabis is close to 10% with a range
extending to over 20%.

Their findings are illustrated in Figure 7.3.

More recent data from the U.K. Government Forensic Science Service were presented to the Advisory Council on the Misuse of Drugs (2005)
(Table 7.8). The data for the period 1995–2005 showed no consistent
changes in the potency of imported cannabis resin, but an upward trend in
the potency of cultivated cannabis.

The conclusion on both sides of the Atlantic seems to be that the
forms of cannabis that have traditionally been available commercially, imported herbal cannabis and cannabis resin, have changed relatively little in
their potency over a period of more than 20 years. However, the increasing
popularity of cannabis from cultivated plants is changing the picture. The
new strains of cannabis have been bred for intensive indoor cultivation,
with plants of short stature and high THC content, and growth conditions
are optimized. They yield herbal cannabis that contains two to three times
more THC than has generally been available previously. Such home-
grown material already accounts for more than half of the cannabis used as

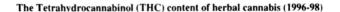

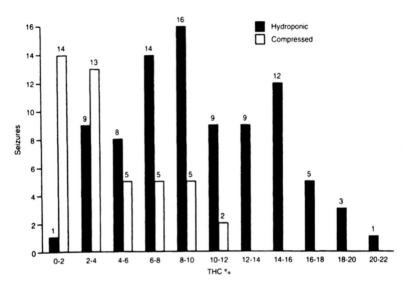

Figure 7.3. Tetrahydrocannabinol content of herbal cannabis samples seized by the police in Britain during the period 1996–1998. Data for imported "compressed" herbal cannabis are shown separately from home-grown "hydroponic" cannabis. (Results provided by the U.K. Forensic Science Service to the House of Lords Cannabis Report, 1998.)

a recreational drug in the United Kingdom and in some other European countries.

But the increase in potency is two- to threefold, not the often quoted 10- to 20-fold. Is the availability of high-potency cannabis products necessarily a matter of concern? Looking at some of the positive aspects, one could argue that if people are going to consume cannabis illegally, then is it not better that they consume material that has been grown under clean conditions? This is more likely than imported cannabis to be free of fungi or other microbial infections and will be less likely to have been adulterated with other potentially toxic materials as commonly happens in imported cannabis resin. Because of the strictly controlled growing conditions, *hydroponic*

Table 7.8. Mean THC Content of Cannabis
Products Seized in the United Kingdom

| Year | Cultivated Cannabis | Imported Resin |
|---|---|---|
| 1995 | 5.8 | No data |
| 1996 | 8.0 | No data |
| 1997 | 9.4 | No data |
| 1998 | 10.5 | 6.1 |
| 1999 | 10.6 | 4.4 |
| 2000 | 12.2 | 4.2 |
| 2001 | 12.3 | 6.7 |
| 2002 | 12.3 | 3.2 |
| 2003 | 12.0 | 4.6 |
| 2004 | 12.7 | 1.6 |
| 2005 | 14.2 | 6.6 |

Data from the Advisory Council on the Misuse of Drugs
(2005), U.K. Forensic Science Service.

*cannabis* will tend to have a highly consistent THC content. Zimmer and
Morgan (1997) rehearsed the arguments for suggesting that high-potency
cannabis may not necessarily lead to an increased intake of THC. Experienced marijuana smokers are able to adjust their smoking behavior to obtain
the desired level of high, and when offered high-potency marijuana they
inhale less smoke (see Chapter 2). From the point of view of the respiratory
system one could argue that high-potency THC is less likely to cause damage to the lungs for this reason, although many users combine cannabis with
tobacco so the benefit of using less cannabis may be small. The fact is that
there has been very little research yet on whether cannabis users change their
behavior when offered a higher potency product, or whether the consumption of skunk or *nederwiet* carries increased health risks or an increased likelihood of dependence. Korf et al. (2004) interviewed 400 visitors to Dutch
coffee shops about the way in which they reacted to the increased potency
of *nederwiet*. They found three types of response: (1) those that stopped
using *nederwiet* because it was too potent; (2) those who inhaled less from
the strong cannabis than from the less potent varieties; and (3) those who
liked to use very strong cannabis and inhaled more. The latter were usually

younger people—and they would clearly be at the greatest risk. But it is too early to know whether such findings will be representative of future trends. Meanwhile, the Netherlands government is sponsoring research to find out empirically whether the high-potency cannabis will change smoking behavior. By analogy with alcohol, the comparison of the higher potency cultivated cannabis with what was previously available is similar to the comparison of wine (10% to 15% alcohol) with beer (3% to 5% alcohol).

It is possible that the availability of these new forms of high-potency marijuana will tempt some users to increase their THC intake, and this in turn could lead to a higher risk of dependency. With any psychoactive drug, it is the users at the upper end of the consumption range who run the greatest risk of dependency.

In summary, the more extravagant claims about superpotent cannabis suggesting that recreational users today are exposed to a wholly different drug from the one their parents may have consumed 20 to 30 years ago are not supported by the evidence. On the other hand, cultivated cannabis is a rapidly growing source of supply and it does contain a considerably higher THC content than has previously been available. Whether this is necessarily dangerous is not clear; it could increase the risk of dependency, but it may also be that the better consistency and quality of this product exposes users to fewer health hazards than previously.

## Is Marijuana a Gateway Drug?

Another widely debated question is whether the use of marijuana leads people to use other illicit drugs, and eventually to become addicted to these. Those who believe this to be true argue that even if marijuana is a relatively harmless drug, it can act as a stepping stone to other far more dangerous drugs.

This is a difficult question to address scientifically. Many surveys have shown that young people who use illegal psychoactive drugs begin with alcohol and tobacco and then marijuana. They tend to experiment with a number of other illicit drugs. Most who take heroin or cocaine will have had previous experience with marijuana and several other illicit substances.

Kandel and Davies (1996), for example, surveyed 7,611 students aged 13 to 18 in 53 New York State schools. Of the total, 995 had experienced marijuana and 403 had experienced cocaine and 121 of these had taken crack cocaine. Alcohol and/or cigarette use tended to begin at age 12 to 13, marijuana use at age 15, and cocaine use at age 15 to 16. The young people who used drugs lived in social environments in which they perceived the use of drugs to be prevalent. Of the students who used crack cocaine, two thirds reported that all or most of their friends had used marijuana and 38% had used cocaine. Among nonusers of drugs, the corresponding figures were 8% and 0%, respectively. But this does not prove that one drug leads to another, as Zimmer and Morgan (1997) point out:

> In the end, the gateway theory is not a theory at all. It is a description of the typical sequence in which multiple drug users initiate the use of high prevalence and low prevalence drugs. A similar statistical relationship exists between other kinds of common and uncommon related activities. For example, most people who ride a motorcycle (a fairly rare activity) have ridden a bicycle (a fairly common activity). Indeed the prevalence of motorcycle riding among people who have never ridden a bicycle is probably extremely low. However, bicycle riding does not cause motorcycle riding, and increases in the former will not lead automatically to increases in the latter. Nor will increases in marijuana use automatically lead to increases in the use of cocaine or other drugs.

Kandel et al. (1996) found that parental behavior was an important determinant of the drug user's behavior. Parental use of alcohol and cigarettes was important in determining experimentation with these drugs. Perhaps more surprisingly, parental use of a medically prescribed tranquilizer was likely to be associated with children's experimentation with illicit drugs. Through their use of legally available psychotropic drugs, parents may indicate to their children that drugs can be used to handle their own feelings of psychological distress.

So is the relationship that does exist between marijuana use and harder drugs simply a matter of social context? Is it the introduction to the underground world of illicit drugs through the black market in marijuana that leads people to experiment with other illicit substances? The Dutch believe that this relationship can be broken by separating the supply of hard drugs from that of marijuana, and making the latter freely available (Chapter 8). The Police Foundation (2000) in their review of the U.K. drug laws found this to be a persuasive argument:

> It seems that Holland can justly claim to have separated the heroin and cannabis markets. As a result, young people are far less likely in Holland than elsewhere to experiment with heroin. Although there is room for argument over precisely how this has been achieved, it is difficult to deny that the policy of separation of markets, including the toleration of coffee shops, has made a contribution.... By doing so the Dutch have provided persuasive evidence against the gateway theory of cannabis use, and in favour of the theory that if there is a gateway it is the illegal market place.

But is there any scientific basis for the gateway theory? Basic research has shown that THC can trigger activity in neural pathways in animal brain that use the chemical messenger dopamine (Fig. 4.2; Chapter 4). The significance of these findings is that this is a common feature seen in response to a variety of addictive central nervous system (CNS) drugs, including alcohol, nicotine, cocaine, amphetamines, and heroin. Some scientists have argued that it is the release of the chemical dopamine in certain key regions of the brain that is responsible for the rewarding effects of these drugs and that leads the user to wish to use them again. Others would argue that this is too simplistic, and that the significance of triggering dopamine release is that it may be getting the brain's attention to some significant stimulus (in this case the psychotropic drug), and that this in turn may helping to determine the animal's motivation for seeking to repeat the experience. Furthermore, since alcohol and nicotine trigger dopamine release in the same way as THC, one could equally well argue that these too should be considered gateway drugs to cocaine, heroin, or amphetamines. The results with THC, however, also show that the effect of THC on dopamine release is apparently due to its ability to trigger a release of naturally occurring opioid substances in the brain (see Chapter 4). There also seems to be some crossover in the dependence syndromes caused by cannabinoids and opioids (Chapter 4). One could suggest that the reason that some people become dependent on cannabis is because they can become addicted to their own naturally occurring opioid chemicals. Using cannabis may prime the brain to seek substances like heroin that act on the same opiate receptors.

Brain researchers now see the endogenous opioid and cannabinoid systems in the CNS as two independent but parallel and overlapping physiological regulatory systems. Both are involved in controlling sensitivity to pain, and both may be involved in some way in reward mechanisms in the brain. But the subjective experience of taking marijuana is quite different from that induced by heroin or other opiate drugs. Experimental animals also find these drugs different; animals trained to discriminate THC or morphine do not generalize to the other drug; and there is no evidence that administering THC makes animals more likely to self-administer heroin. The neurobiological basis for the gateway theory is speculative at best.

## Do Recreational Marijuana Users Become Dependent?

Chapter 4 discussed how drug dependence (formerly called *addiction*) can be assessed by using an internationally agreed-upon standard psychiatric questionnaire—the DSM-IV—and reviewed basis research in animals that shows THC to be capable of inducing dependence. But how serious a problem is this for recreational users of cannabis?

Wayne Hall and Nadia Solowij, internationally recognized experts in the field of addiction research, described how they view this situation:

> Dependence on cannabis is the most prevalent and under-appreciated risk of regular cannabis users. About 10% of those who ever use cannabis, and one third to one half of those who use it daily will lose control over their cannabis use and continue to use the drug in the face of problems they believe are caused or exacerbated by its use....Uncertainty remains as to how difficult it is to overcome cannabis dependence and what is the best way to assist individuals to become abstinent. (Hall and Solowij, 1997)

Dr. Hall in testimony to the House of Lords enquiry (1998) said:

> By popular repute, cannabis is not a drug of dependence because it does not have a clearly defined withdrawal syndrome. There is, however, little doubt that some users who want to stop or cut down their cannabis use find it very difficult to do so, and continue to use cannabis despite the adverse effects that it has on their lives.... Epidemiological studies suggest that cannabis dependence in the sense of impaired control over use is the most common form of drug dependence after tobacco and alcohol, affecting as many as one in ten of those who ever use the drug.

A survey of more than 10,000 people in Australia, where heavy use if cannabis is common, reported that 20% of the cannabis users in this group met DSM-IV criteria for substance dependence (Swift et al., 2001). In the United States a survey of more than 40,000 adults in 1991–1992 showed that 4% reported using cannabis during the past year, and of these 7.5% were diagnosed as dependent; by 2001–2002 in a similar survey the rate of cannabis use remained the same but the proportion of dependent users had risen to 10%.

In some people the drug will come to dominate their life. They will feel a psychological need and craving for the drug, and will become preoccupied with locating continuing supplies of the drug. Consumption of marijuana may become so frequent that the user remains almost permanently stoned. They may prepare a joint before going to sleep at night in order to ensure that it is available for the morning. The severely dependent user is permanently cognitively impaired, lacks motivation, tends to suffer from lowered self-esteem, may be depressed, and is unlikely to be able to function at all in work or education. Although most regular cannabis users suffer merely mild discomfort when they stop taking the drug, the severely dependent user will suffer a definite syndrome of unpleasant withdrawal symptoms—including anxiety, depression, sleep disturbance, nausea, and loose stools or diarrhea. Cannabis dependence is still largely unrecognized, because many users continue to believe that it is not an addictive drug. There is a real need to educate cannabis users, to convey the message that they do run a risk of allowing the drug to dominate their lives.

The DSM-IV definition of dependence, however, is only a label—you are either "dependent" or "not dependent," although the DSM does allow for a lesser category of "substance abuse." But in reality there are many degrees of dependence, as shown clearly by a detailed analysis of the wide variety of symptoms reported by 1,474 cannabis users in the United States (Denton and Earlywine, 2006). Among the whole population of cannabis users there is probably a continuous gradation from harmless weekend users to the problem heavy users whose severe dependence may wreck their lives.

If one attempts to assess the risk of dependence by comparison to other addictive drugs, cannabis does not score top of the list in terms of either the severity of the addiction or the likelihood of becoming hooked. The Institute of Medicine (1999) report suggested that 9% of those who ever used cannabis become dependent (as defined by the DSM criteria); this compared with dependency risks of 32% for tobacco, 23% for heroin, 17% for cocaine, and 15% for alcohol. Cocaine and heroin are far more damaging, both in terms of the severity of the physical withdrawal syndrome that users will experience if they stop taking the drug and in the probability of becoming hooked on the drug. Nicotine is notorious in the sense that a very high proportion of cigarette smokers tend to become permanent smokers after consuming only a few packs of cigarettes (Kozlowski et al., 1989). Unlike the casual user of marijuana, the cigarette smoker typically smokes 15 to 20 a day every day of the year. Unlike cigarette smokers, most marijuana smokers also seem to be able to give up the habit relatively easily. As they reach their 30s and become responsible for a family and a job, many are no longer willing to take the risk of being punished for illegal drug use, although as noted previously this pattern may change as the drug-wise baby boomer generation ages.

Another way of measuring the extent of cannabis dependence is to ask how many people seek treatment for it. In Britain, Department of Health figures for 1996 showed that in 6% of all contacts with regional drug clinics cannabis was the main drug of abuse, but these numbers have doubled in the past 10 years. In Australia the numbers seeking treatment for cannabis have more than tripled since 1992, and represent 21% of all those seeking treatment for drug dependence. In the United States the Department of

Health and Human Services reported a fivefold increase in those seeking treatment for cannabis abuse in the period 1992–2001. In Ontario, Canada, in 2000–2001 38% of those seeking treatment for drug dependence cited cannabis as a concern, and 13% cited it as the primary problem. These are alarming statistics, which at first sight suggest that cannabis dependence is a fast-growing problem, perhaps in part as a consequence of the increased use of very high-potency cannabis products. This may be partly true, but there are other factors at work. In some countries, notably in the United States and Canada, treatment is frequently offered as an alternative to criminal punishment for minor possession offenses, or as a result of testing positive in the workplace. In Ontario 38% of those who cited cannabis as their primary problem also reported that they were under external pressure to seek treatment. To what extent the U.S. figures are inflated by people on compulsory treatment is impossible to disentangle.

There is little doubt that cannabis dependence is a problem, and it is likely to grow. Unfortunately, there have been very few controlled trials to assess treatment methods, which remain mainly focused on group counseling. There are no effective medications to assist the dependent cannabis user, although the antagonist rimonabant is an obvious candidate to prevent relapse if not to treat craving, in the same way as the opiate antagonist naltrexone is used in treating opiate dependence. (For review see Roffman and Stephens, 2006.)

## Forensic Testing for Cannabis—Growth Industry

Cannabis is a potent drug, so the concentrations of THC and THC metabolites in blood or other body fluids are very low. Whereas alcohol is present in quite high concentrations and is thus easy to measure in blood or breath, measuring cannabis proved technically much more difficult. Until the 1980s THC could only be measured in blood or urine samples after concentrating the sample and using complex chromatography equipment. The problem was solved by the development of immunoassay kits. These depend on using THC or its major metabolite to stimulate the immune system of animals to produce antibodies that recognize THC or the metabolite carboxy-THC (Fig. 2.6). Antibodies recognize the compounds at very low concentrations, and they can be used as reagents in tests that involve measuring the binding of THC or carboxy-THC that triggers a change in fluorescence, triggers a color reaction, or displaces a radioactive tracer. The availability of commercial kits for cannabis testing in urine has made such testing widespread. It is now routine to test road accident victims and hospital emergency room admissions for cannabis and a range of other psychoactive drugs. The finding that a significant proportion of people involved in road traffic accidents or admitted to hospital emergency rooms are cannabis positive has been given much publicity, but this ignores the fact that the use of cannabis is widespread, and since the tests yield positive results for pharmacologically inactive THC metabolites for long periods after the last drug use, it is not surprising to find many people registering positive. Drug testing in the workplace and schools has also become common—particularly in the United States. Here the consequences of testing positive for cannabis can often be severe—enroll in a cannabis treatment program and stop using the drug or be expelled from school or lose your job. Civil rights lawyers have questioned the ethics and legality of punishing someone for use of cannabis in their own free time, without any ability to distinguish drug use from drug abuse.

Because of the long persistence of THC in the body, cannabis tests fail to give a reliable indication of the state of intoxication of the user. A urine concentration of 50 ng/ml for carboxy-THC is generally taken as the definition of a positive test. Such levels may occur in urine for days or even weeks after the last dose of drug. By measuring the ratio of carboxy-THC to unchanged THC, some idea can be obtained of how long ago the last dose was taken—since this ratio increases with time. These measurements, though, do not have the same value as measurements of alcohol in breath or blood—which give a far more accurate picture of the state of intoxication of the drinker at that moment. A recent improvement using antibody methodology allows testing for THC in saliva (http://www.cozart.biz). This has the advantage of offering a direct measure of recent cannabis consumption, and is thus a meaningful way of assessing, for example, whether a driver was intoxicated. A mobile kit allows police to use this as a roadside test. Forensic testing with new techniques of gas chromatography linked to mass spectroscopy gives an even more sensitive method for detecting minute quantities of THC—levels of 1 ng/ml or less can readily be measured. These techniques can be applied to the analysis of the drug in hair samples—thus giving a picture of whether an individual has used the drug over extended periods of time, information that could be valuable to assess compliance with treatment programs.

## Snapshots of Cannabis Use Around the World

Cannabis has been used for hundreds of years in different countries and cultures, both for recreational and medicinal uses and as an integral part of religious rites (for reviews see Rubin, 1975; Robinson, 1996; and Booth, 2003). An understanding of this may help us to place the modern vogue for cannabis use in the Western world into a broader context. Many modern users of cannabis speak of their feelings of spirituality and "oneness with God" when intoxicated. Cannabis is used in many religions as a sacrament, from the dagga cults in Africa to the Ethiopian Copts, Hindus, Zoroastrians, Rastas, Buddhists, Taoists, and Sufis. Unlike drinking alcohol, the use of cannabis is not expressly forbidden in the Koran, and in some Moslem countries cannabis tends to take the place filled by alcohol elsewhere.

### India and Pakistan

The report of the Indian Hemp Drugs Commission (1894) gave a detailed account of the use of cannabis in the Indian subcontinent more than 100 years ago (see Chapter 8), and Chopra and Chopra (1957) described a situation that seemed to have changed little almost half a century later. There are two principal methods of consuming cannabis. Dried herbal cannabis, known as *bhang*, may be chewed or eaten, or more commonly used to make a beverage often known as *thandai*. Many variants of this drink exist; bhang may be mixed with many other ingredients including milk, almonds, melon and poppy seeds, aniseed, cardamons, musk, and essence of rose. Sweetmeats containing bhang and even ice cream containing the powdered leaves may also be used. Whereas alcohol is generally looked down upon in Hindu society, high-caste Hindus are allowed bhang at religious ceremonials, and also employ it as an intoxicant at marriage ceremonies and family festivals. Bhang is used traditionally by laborers in India in much the same way as beer is used in the United States. A few pulls at a ganja pipe or a glass of bhang at the end of the day relieves fatigue and provides them with a sense of well-being, to enable them to bear more cheerfully the strain and monotony of their daily routines. Bhang is used in the Hindu religion in particular to celebrate the last day of the Durga Puja, and offerings are made to the god Shiva in Hindu temples. Bhang is also used by itinerant Hindu ascetics:

> Fulfilling a spiritual function…, the ascetics—called sadhus—radiate spiritual energy as they walk about the country, feeding the consciousness of India and the planet, and believe that the use of bhang supplies them with spiritual power, brings them closer to enlightenment, and honors Shiva, who is said to be perpetually intoxicated by cannabis.
> Voluntarily homeless, the sadhus live in the forest or in caves or walk perpetually, subsisting on alms. Their hair hangs in long matted strands, their skin is covered with dust or ashes, and they wear only a few rags or nothing at all. Sadhus practice physical austerities including celibacy and long fasts without food or water. Bhang is said to help them center their thoughts on the divine and to endure hardships. (Robinson, 1996)

The widespread use of bhang, however, has decreased markedly in modern India. Bhang is probably equivalent to low-grade marijuana in its THC content, and the watery infusions that are drunk probably contain rather little active drug, although milk (which contains fats) would be a more effective means of extracting THC. Intoxication after taking bhang is uncommon, and the Indian Hemp Drugs Commission's conclusion in 1897 that the moderate use of hemp drugs caused no appreciable physical, mental, or moral injury was probably correct. The other method of consumption, smoking *ganja* (the compressed female flower heads) or *charas* (cannabis resin), commonly in an earthware pipe known as a *chillum*, doubtless delivers more active drug. Smoking is always a communal activity, involving two to five people. Workmen, fishermen, farmers, and others who had to work long hours smoked cannabis to alleviate fatigue and relive physical stress, often at the end of a working day, and sportsmen took it to improve their physical strength and endurance. Intoxication was rare, and most users were able to carry on their work or other activities. Ganja and charas smoking was generally looked down upon by the middle classes as a working class activity.

## Nepal and Tibet

The advent of the hippie era and the migration of young Westerners to the Himalayas in search of cannabis and spiritual enlightenment led to some remarkable changes in local attitudes to cannabis in these cultures. In Nepal cannabis was traditionally used by Hindu yogis as an aid to meditation, and male devotees used it as a symbol of fellowship in their communal consumption of the drug. It was also used by older people to while away the time when they were too old to work in the fields. The advent of the hippie era and an influx of Westerners, however, brought about increased cultivation of cannabis, inflated prices, and a change in attitude of young, middle-class Nepalese to the extent that smoking cannabis came to be regarded as a novel, acceptable, and pleasurable mark of sophistication. This in turn led a panic-stricken government in Nepal to introduce harsh new laws during the 1970s in an attempt to suppress the use of the drug (Rubin, 1975).

In Tibet cannabis plays a significant role in some Buddhist ceremonies. According to Indian tradition and writings, Siddhartha used and ate nothing but hemp and its seeds for 6 years prior to announcing his truths and becoming the Buddha in the fifth century BC.

## Southeast Asia

Cannabis is common in Cambodia, Thailand, Laos, and Vietnam—many Americans were introduced for the first time to the drug during military service in Vietnam in the 1960s and 1970s. The plant tends to be cultivated on a family basis, with a few plants growing around the house. Herbal cannabis is freely available in markets, and is smoked together with tobacco. The herbal material is also used extensively in the local cuisine to impart an agreeable flavor and mild euphoriant quality. Medically, cannabis is recognized as a pain reliever and in the treatment of cholera, malaria, dysentery, asthma, and convulsions. Cannabis is considered to be a source of social well-being, to be shared with friends, and is also used to ease difficult work tasks (see Rubin, 1975).

## Africa

The use of cannabis both for pleasure and for religious purposes is common throughout most of Africa, where it predates the arrival of Europeans. Known commonly as *dagga*, cannabis is a sacrament and a medicine to the Pygmies, Zulus, and Hottentots. Its use in religious ceremonies in Ethiopia is ancient, and it was taken up and used as a sacrament there by the early Coptic Christian church.

In Morocco cannabis, known as *kif*, is traditionally served as a stimulant and as a means of relieving the pressures of daily life among the tribal groups living in the Rif Mountains. The growing of cannabis in this Northern region of the country has become an important agricultural export industry for an area that was previously the poorest agricultural area. In Morocco and other countries in North Africa many people maintain special rooms where kif is smoked while traditional stories, dances, and songs are passed on to the young generation.

## Caribbean and Latin America

Jamaica has become an important cultivation center for cannabis. The drug, known as ganja, was brought there by laborers from India in the midnineteenth century and spread to the black working class community, where its use has become widespread. Ganja smoking is so prevalent among working-class males that the nonsmoker is regarded as a deviant. The occasion of first smoking attains the cultural significance of an initiation rite, and ideally should be accompanied by the *ganja vision*. Jamaica is also the home of a twentieth-century religion known as Rastifarianism founded by Marcus Garvey in the 1930s, in which cannabis plays a key role. Members of this religion, known as Rastas, accept some parts of the Bible, but believe

that the Ethiopian Emperor Haile Selassie was a living God and represented "Jesus for the black race." Ethiopia is thought of as the ancient place
of origin of black people, and an eventual return to Ethiopia would be their
equivalent of nirvana. The ritual smoking of cannabis forms a key part of
the Rastifarian religion; it is thought to cleanse both body and mind, preparing the user for prayer and meditation. Rastas, with their characteristic
dreadlocks and their dedication to cannabis, have permeated many aspects
of modern culture, especially in the field of pop music. One of the most
famous was the musician Bob Marley, who died in 1981. In a song entitled
*Kaya* written in 1978 he sang openly about marijuana (*kaya* is a Jamaican
street term for marijuana):

> Wake up and turn I loose
> Wake up and turn I loose
> For the rain is falling

> Got to have kaya now, got to have kaya now
> Got to have kaya now, for the rain is falling

> I feel so high, I even touch the sky
> Above the falling rain
> I feel so good in my neighborhood
> So here I come again

The Zion Coptic Church is an American sect modeled on the Rastifarian movement in Jamaica; it too maintains a cannabis-based Eucharist. In
1989 Carl Olsen, a member of this church, sought to gain exemption from
the cannabis prohibition laws in the United States by claiming the rights of
church members under the First Amendment of the American Constitu-
tion to have the freedom to pursue their own religion, which in this case
required the use of marijuana as a sacrament. The U.S. Drug Enforcement
Agency won the case, pointing out among other things that Olsen's action
in importing 20 tons of marijuana into the country seemed suspicious, as
this was an outrageously large quantity to supply the few hundred members
of the church in the United States. One of those involved, Jim Tranmer,
was later jailed for 35 years, protesting of religious persecution.

Cannabis smoking is common in many Latin American countries. Sometimes, as in Brazil, it was brought there by African slaves and spread among the working people as "the opium of the poor." In Mexico and Colombia the cultivation of cannabis for export has become an important cash crop, and along with this has come a widespread use of the drug. Whereas marijuana smoking in Colombia was formerly regarded as socially undesirable, it has become acceptable in many circles. Mexico has been the home of a number of religious sects that use cannabis as a sacrament. For example, a small community near the Gulf of Mexico uses marijuana, which they call *la santa rosa*, in their religious ceremonies. The dried herbal cannabis rests on the divine altar wrapped in small bundles of paper, along with artefacts of ancient local gods and images of Catholic saints. The men and women priests of the church chew small quantities of the herb and it gives them inspiration to preach to the congregation. The French anthropologist Louis Livet (1920) described a remarkable communal marijuana ritual among a sect of native Indians in Mexico. Participants were seated in a circle and each in turn took a puff at a large marijuana cigar, which he then passed to his neighbor. The atmosphere at such meetings was joyful and filled with ritual chanting and convivial warmth. Each of those attending took a total of 13 puffs, and at the end consequently found himself in state of hallucinatory excitement and intoxication. At the center of the circle was placed a sacred animal, an iguana. The animal, attracted by the smell of the marijuana smoke, also rotated 13 times, turning its head towards the cigar with its mouth open, inhaling the smoke. The animal was thought to represent the sacred incarnation of a god presiding over the ceremony, and when the iguana became intoxicated and fell down, the participants knew that it was time to stop passing the cigar! The reptile served a function akin to that of the pit canary in nineteenth century coal mines!

## Conclusions

The recreational use of cannabis has become common in most Western countries. As of now it is an activity indulged in mainly those under the age of 30, but this pattern may change as cannabis becomes more and more accepted as part of our culture. It has been accepted and widely used, often as an alternative to alcohol, in many parts of the world.

There are health risks associated with cannabis use, particularly with smoked marijuana, but earlier reports of the dangers of cannabis have proved to be exaggerated. There is a genuine risk of developing dependence on cannabis, and for some people it can come to dominate their lives and have a very negative impact. To many people it is regarded, rightly or wrongly, as a harmless weekend indulgence.

# 8

*What Next?*
*A Hundred Years of*
*Cannabis Reports*

I t is not the purpose of this book to persuade the reader to join one side or the other of the cannabis wars, but rather to seek some middle ground in this debate, which has become so polarized. By writing a book that attempts to take a cautious attitude to the limited scientific facts known about the subject, the author already invites the criticism levied against Wayne Hall et al. (1994) for their balanced review of *The Health and Psychological Consequences of Cannabis Use* prepared for the Australian government that they were guilty of "harmful caution" (Ghodse, 1996). As Dr. Ghodse put it:

> The authors have been rigorous in making sure that their inferences are largely based on established evidence. This high degree of caution in interpreting evidence is commendable but has led to salient information on the probable health consequences of cannabis use that should be succinctly transmissible to the public, being diluted. This in turn has led to the presentation of an optimistic view of the consequences of cannabis use that renders the authors' apparent caution prejudicial, or even harmful.

By the beginning of the new millennium we reached an interesting stage in the cannabis debate in the Western world. We must soon decide whether to reintroduce it into our medicine cabinets and whether to accept, albeit reluctantly, that the recreational use of cannabis has become part of our culture. There are even the first stirrings of a debate about the legalization or *decriminalization* of cannabis. Can we learn something from the many reviews of these subjects that have been sponsored by governments and other bodies during the past century?

Cannabis was made illegal almost by accident. It was added to the agenda of the League of Nations 1925 Convention on Narcotic Control because Egypt and Turkey proposed it. The Egyptian delegate denounced *hashism*, which he claimed caused 30% to 60% of the insanity in his country. Hashish addicts, he said, were regarded as useless derelicts. With little opposition, and no attempt to verify these claims, 57 nations signed the Convention banning cannabis. The United States did not sign this Convention, but American newspapers in the 1920s and 1930s ran many stories about "colored" men crazed with marijuana allegedly carrying big knives and prone to extreme violence and rape. Henry Anslinger, head of the Federal Bureau of Narcotics, organized a vigorous campaign against "demon dope" using films and posters, associating cannabis with jazz ("voodoo music"), interracial sex, madness, and death. In 1937 the U.S. Marijuana Tax Act effectively made cannabis illegal.

## A Hundred Years of Cannabis Inquiries

A cynic might suggest that the decision to hold an expert enquiry into cannabis is the politician's way of avoiding having to debate the issue or to take any action. There have been a number of expert enquiries around the world; nearly all have concluded that cannabis is a remarkably safe drug and many have recommended that limited medical use be permitted pending the outcome of the more detailed clinical research that is needed to approve properly sanctioned cannabis-based medicines. None of these enquiries led to any substantial legislative changes until very recently. Some of the more important ones are worth considering.

### The Indian Hemp Drugs Commission Report (1894)

For long this was an obscure document, but it has rightly been given a new lease of life in recent years. This is a remarkable example of the manner in which the British Empire was governed in the nineteenth century. As Britain expanded her empire in India there was concern that the abuse of cannabis by the native people might be endangering their health. There were rumors that the asylums in India were filling with those driven insane by the abuse of cannabis. The late nineteenth century saw the British Parliament finally abolish the slave trade and put in place new restrictions on the consumption of opium and alcohol in Britain. The Temperance League was formed to combat the evils of alcohol. One of the leaders of that movement raised a question in the British Parliament in March 1893 querying the morality of the trade in cannabis in India, a trade that was not only sanctioned by the British Indian administration, but that also provided

substantial tax revenues. The British government requested the government of India:

> ... to appoint a Commission to inquire into the cultivation of the hemp plant
> in Bengal, the preparation of drugs from it, the trade in these drugs, the effect
> of their consumption upon the social and moral condition of the people, and
> the desirability of prohibiting the growth of the plant and the sale of ganja
> and allied drugs.

The Commission consisting of eminent British and Indian administra-
tors and medical experts reviewed the situation not just in Bengal but in all
of British India. They undertook interviews with a total of 1,193 witnesses in
13 different provinces or cities, using a standardized series of questions. The
witnesses were carefully chosen to represent both officials and a wide range
of citizens; they were asked about the cultivation of hemp in their region,
the preparation and consumption of hemp-related drugs, and the effects
that the consumption of these were thought to have on the physical and
moral well-being of the users. A particular question that the Commission
addressed was whether or not the consumption of cannabis led to insanity,
as claimed by some. All of the mental asylums in British India were visited and the records of every patient claimed to be suffering from cannabis-
induced psychosis carefully examined. The conclusion was that in most
cases cannabis could not be held responsible, and in the few genuine cases
of cannabis-induced psychosis the illness proved to be short lived and re-
versible on stopping the use of the drug. This conclusion is consistent with
what most contemporary psychiatrists now believe. After 2 years of detailed
and thorough work, the Commission published its conclusions and the supporting data in a six-volume document in 1894. Its conclusions concerning
herbal cannabis (*bhang*) can be summarized as follows (see Chapter 6):

> The Commission are prepared to state that the suppression of the use of
> bhang would be totally unjustifiable. It is established to their satisfaction that
> this use is very ancient, and that it has some religious sanction among a large
> body of Hindus; that it enters into their social customs; that it is almost with-
> out exception harmless in moderation, and perhaps in some cases beneficial;
> that the abuse of it is not so harmful as the abuse of alcohol...

The Commissioners were more circumspect about the smoked forms of cannabis, ganja and charas (Chapter 1). Several witnesses referred to the habit-forming properties of the smoked drug, a habit that was easy to form but hard to break. The Commission, however, did not feel that prohibition was justified or necessary. Prohibition would in any case be difficult to enforce, would provoke an outcry from religious users, and might stimulate the use of other more dangerous narcotics.

In addition, there was the question of what to do about alcohol:

> Apart from all this, there is another consideration which has been urged in some quarters with a manifestation of strong feeling, and to which the Commission are disposed to attach some importance, viz, that to repress the hemp drugs in India and to leave alcohol alone would be misunderstood by a large number of persons who believe, and apparently not without reason, that more harm is done in this country by the latter than by the former.

The Commission's report is remarkably sophisticated and surprisingly relevant to many of the issues debated in the present-day cannabis wars. The fact that several of the cannabis-producing regions of India received a significant part of their local government income from the revenues imposed by the British on the trade in cannabis products may have influenced the Commission's benign conclusions, but it remains a thorough and objective analysis.

## Mayor La Guardia's Report, *The Marihuana Problem in the City of New York* (1944)

Despite the passing of the Cannabis Tax Act in 1937, the illicit consumption of cannabis continued to grow in American cities, and it gained a notorious reputation in the media as a "killer drug," a view encouraged by Harry Anslinger. In New York Mayor La Guardia decided to try to find out just how harmful cannabis was. He appointed a committee of scientists to investigate, and the resulting investigation was the most thorough since the Indian Hemp Drugs Commission 50 years earlier. The committee organized clinical research on the effects of marijuana, using 77 prison volunteers (it was common practice at the time to use such volunteers as research subjects; most American pharmaceutical companies, for example, tested their new medicines on prisoners). The volunteers were given large doses of a cannabis extract or were allowed to smoke marijuana during a period of up to 1 month while in the Welfare Island Hospital. The doses of tetrahydrocannabinol (THC) were unknown, but must have been quite high since almost all the subjects became high even at the lowest of the doses administered. The researchers were impressed with the low incidence of adverse side effects. The most common were anxiety (particularly among those subjects who had not used the drug before), nausea and vomiting, and ataxia (clumsiness). Nine subjects reported what were referred to as psychotic episodes, but these were all transient and were not considered serious. In addition, a careful comparison was made between a group of 60 prisoners on Ward's Island who had been daily marijuana smokers with a similar number of nonusers. The investigators concluded:

> Prolonged use of the drug does not lead to physical, mental or moral degeneration, nor have we observed any permanent deleterious effects from its continued use.

As important as the clinical studies was the sociological research commissioned by the committee, using police officers in civilian clothes who lived in the areas of the city in which marijuana use and peddling were common. The question of how widespread marijuana use was among school children was also addressed. The investigators concluded that marijuana use was largely confined to the poorer communities in the city, particularly in Harlem; that there was no link between marijuana use and crime; and that the drug did not provoke violent behavior. There was no evidence of widespread use among school children. Furthermore, the report concluded:

> We have been unable to confirm the opinion expressed by some investigators that marijuana smoking is the first step in the use of such drugs as cocaine, morphine and heroin. The instances are extremely rare where the habit of marijuana smoking is associated with addiction to these other narcotics.

But although Mayor La Guardia's (1944) report was one of the clearest and most thorough investigations ever undertaken, its conclusions did not make much impression on public opinion in America at the time. The conclusion that marijuana was a relatively harmless drug was not what the media or Harry Anslinger wanted to hear. Anslinger was vehemently opposed to cannabis, and he was harshly critical of the report's conclusions, labeling them as "giddy sociology, and medical mumbo-jumbo." Even the influential *Journal of the American Medical Association* attacked the report in an editorial, which concluded:

> Public officials will do well to disregard this unscientific, uncritical study and continue to regard marijuana as a menace wherever it is purveyed.

Jerome Himmelstein (1978) in his book *The Strange Career of Marihuana* gives some remarkable insights into the strange history of the politics and ideology of cannabis in the United States. Detailed accounts of this history can also be found in Abel (1943), Robinson (1996), Bonnie and Whitbread (1974), Booth (2003), and Russo (2007). Public perceptions of the drug owed little to a dispassionate review of the scientific facts and much more to the dedicated anti-cannabis crusade of Harry Anslinger and his Federal Bureau of Narcotics and the popular disapproval of marijuana as a drug associated with the lower classes and with Mexican immigrants.

## *The Wootton Report*, England (1969)

The widespread consumption of cannabis did not begin in England or in most West European countries until the 1960s. Attitudes to the control of the drug until then were driven largely by events across the Atlantic and by the various international agreements that were put into place, starting with the League of Nations in 1925 and the subsequent World Health Organization Single Convention on Narcotic Drugs adopted in 1964, which similarly categorized cannabis as a Schedule I drug of addiction with no medical uses.

It was only when the use of cannabis suddenly expanded in the 1960s that the government of the time felt any need to take it more seriously. The British Home Office, in charge of the regulation of illicit drugs, established a group of experts known as the Advisory Committee on Drug Dependence, and an expert subcommittee of this was set up "to review available evidence on the pharmacological, clinical, pathological, social and legal aspects of these drugs (cannabis and lysergic acid)." An experienced sociologist and politician, Baroness Wootton, chaired the subcommittee. While the subcommittee was deliberating, an advertisement appeared in the *Times* newspaper on the July 24, 1967, asserting that the dangers of cannabis use had been exaggerated and advocating a relaxation of the laws governing its consumption. This provoked a wave of hostile debate in the media and in Parliament. The *Wootton Report*, as the document submitted to the Home Secretary, James Callaghan, in 1968 became known, made a big impact (Advisory Committee on Drug Dependence, 1969). Its conclusions were clear:

> We think that the adverse effects which the consumption of cannabis in even small amounts may produce in some people should not be dismissed as insignificant. We have no doubt that the wider use of cannabis should not be encouraged. On the other hand, we think that the dangers of its use as commonly accepted in the past and the risk of progressing to opiates have been overstated, and that the existing criminal sanctions intended to curb its use are unjustifiably severe.

The report went on to recommend a number of changes to the criminal law, the chief of which would have made the possession of small amounts of cannabis for personal use no longer an imprisonable offense, but merely punishable by a summary fine. In addition, it recommended that preparations of cannabis should continue to be available for medical uses. But like the La Guardia report earlier, the *Wootton Report* was assailed in the press and parliament as a "charter for drug seekers." By the late 1960s the large-scale spread of cannabis use on both sides of the Atlantic to middle-class youth altered public perceptions of the problem. Cannabis use had become a symbol in the public mind of the hippie counterculture and the increasing alienation of young people from society. Perhaps these considerations lead the British Home Secretary James Callaghan to criticize the report even before it had been officially released, and in a statement to Parliament shortly after the publication of the report he said:

> I think it came as a surprise, if not a shock, to most people, when that notorious advertisement appeared in the Times in 1967, to find that there is a

lobby in favour of legalising cannabis.... It is another aspect of the so-called permissive society, and I am glad if my decision has enabled the House to call a halt to the advancing tide of permissiveness.

Not only did the Callaghan government ignore the recommendations made in the *Wootton Report*, but also the Misuse of Drugs Act 1971 passed a few years later increased the criminal penalties associated with cannabis use.

## Report Followed Report

At about the same time as the *Wootton Report* was published in England, the U.S. Department of Health Education and Welfare launched an ongoing study of implications of marijuana use in the United States through a National Commission on Marihuana and Drug Abuse. The first of a series of reports, entitled *Marihuana: A Signal of Misunderstanding* (National Commission on Marihuana and Drug Abuse, 1972) (sometimes referred to as the Shafer Commission Report), produced a great impact. It went even further than the *Wootton Report* in recommending that the private possession or distribution of small quantities of cannabis for personal use should no longer be an offense, and that possession in public of up to 1 ounce (28 g) be punishable by a fine of $100.

> Marihuana use is not such a grave problem that individuals who smoke marihuana, and possess it for that purpose, should be subject to criminal prosecution.

Predictably, President Nixon summarily rejected these recommendations and there was a hostile reaction from many other quarters. One year later the Commission published a second report, *Drug Use in America: Problem in Perspective* (National Commission on Marihuana and Drug Abuse, 1973), which backtracked on the earlier recommendations:

> The risk potential of marihuana is quite low compared to the potent psychoactive substances, and even its widespread consumption does not involve the social cost now associated with most of the stimulants and depressants.... Nonetheless, the Commission remains persuaded that availability of this

drug should not be institutionalised at this time.... It is painfully clear from
the debate over our recommendations that the absence of a criminal penalty
is presently equated in too many minds with approval, regardless of a continued prohibition on availability. The Commission regrets that marihuana's
symbolism remains so powerful, obstructing the emergence of a rational
policy.

In Canada the *La Dain Report* (Canadian Government Commission
of Inquiry into the Non-Medical Use of Drugs, 1970) provided a detailed
review of cannabis use and it too recommended a repeal of the prohibition
against the simple possession of cannabis. The Canadian authors also concluded that there was little evidence that cannabis was a drug of addiction.
Like other reports published at that time the Canadian Commission found
little to worry about:

> On the whole, the physical and mental effects of cannabis, at the levels of
> use presently attained in North America, would appear to be much less seri-
> ous than those which may result from excessive use of alcohol.

In Australia and New Zealand, a report on Drug Trafficking and Drug
Abuse published in 1971 revealed that cannabis use was increasing rapidly
in that part of the world, with its favorable climate for cannabis cultivation.
The authors did not appear to be alarmed by this, and recommended that
first-time offenders no longer be subject to prison sentences but be given
suspended fines.

The early 1970s represented the zenith of acceptance of marijuana
as a relatively safe drug. The various groups of experts around the world
who reviewed the subject helped to demolish the commonly held view
that cannabis was a highly dangerous drug that rapidly produced disastrous
effects on the mental and physical health of users. For a while in the 1970s
it looked as if the decriminalization of cannabis might be approved in the
United States and elsewhere around the world. President Jimmy Carter
was reported to be in favor of decriminalization and to have said that:

> Penalties against a drug should not be more dangerous to an individual than
> the use of the drug itself, and where they are they should be changed. (Zim-
> mer and Morgan, 1997)

But it was to be another 30 years before any changes in the legal status of cannabis were seriously considered. During the late 1970s and 1980s, an active anti-marijuana movement gained ground, particularly in the United States. The arguments against the drug were largely moral, and were lead by politicians and by those scientists and psychiatrists who were willing to portray only the adverse effects of the drug. Professor Gabrial Nahas, a scientist at New York University, was a particularly vocal and unashamedly biased campaigner against cannabis. His books *Marihuana—Deceptive Weed* (1973) and *Keep Off the Grass* (1976) helped to inflame if not to illuminate the debate. This campaign was joined also by well-meaning and well-organized groups of middle-class parents who had no direct experience of cannabis but feared the dangers it might hold for their children. The National Institute on Drug Abuse also became more and more actively involved in publicizing the dangers of cannabis use, and continues to do so today (Zimmer and Morgan, 1997).

In the United States and most other countries in the Western world an impasse was reached. Criminal sanctions prohibiting the use of cannabis remained in place, although this seemed to have relatively little effect on the consumption of the drug, which continued to involve increasing numbers of young people. Cannabis was also finally excluded altogether from any medical uses, although as described earlier it was the revival of interest in this aspect of the drug that has rekindled the cannabis debate in recent years.

There have been several more recent reviews of the physical and mental consequences of cannabis use, including the excellent and thorough review by Wayne Hall and colleagues for the Australian government, *The Health and Psychological Consequences of Cannabis Use* (Hall et al., 1994). Most recent was the World Health Organization (WHO) report, *Cannabis: A Health Perspective and Research Agenda* (WHO, 1997). But these reviews largely depended on research done in the 1960s and 1970s— the field of cannabis research was relatively dormant during the 1980s. It came alive again in the 1990s with the new scientific discoveries of cannabinoid receptors and endogenous cannabinoids and the increasing interest in the medical applications of cannabis.

## The Dutch Experiment

Only one country in the West, Holland, decided to decriminalize cannabis. For the past 30 years the Dutch have taken a radically different approach in their drugs policy (for review see Engelsman, 1989). The Netherlands signed the UN Single Convention on Narcotic Drugs (1964) and Dutch law states unequivocally that cannabis is illegal. Yet in 1976 the Dutch adopted a formal policy of nonenforcement for violations involving possession or sale of small quantities of cannabis (originally 30 g, reduced to 5 g since 1995). A series of coffee shops were licensed to sell small quantities of herbal cannabis or cannabis resin for consumption on the premises or to take away. The number of such establishments was small, however, until the late 1980s and 1990s. At their peak more than 1,500 such establishments existed in the Netherlands. They must not hold more than 500 g cannabis in stock, are not permitted to sell alcohol or any other psychoactive drugs, must not cause a nuisance to neighbors, cannot advertise, and are not permitted to sell cannabis to minors. These regulations are strictly policed and licenses can be revoked and the owners punished for violating them. The aims of Dutch drug policy are pragmatic rather than moralistic; they hope to achieve harm reduction by regulating the traffic in cannabis and separating this from the sources of supplies of other illegal and potentially more harmful psychoactive drugs. A Dutch saying can sum up this attitude:

We don't solve a problem by making it taboo and pushing it underground.

But have the objectives of Dutch cannabis policy been achieved? Many critics from outside the country portray lurid tales of decadence and cannabis-doped youth. What are the facts? Did the levels of cannabis use increase rapidly after decriminalization in 1976? Are the levels of cannabis use higher in the Netherlands than in other Western countries? The best available comparisons of data on cannabis consumption among 18- to 20-year-olds show that the new policy had surprisingly little impact on cannabis consumption among young people in Holland, which remained stable for some years after the new policy was introduced until it started to rise in the mid-1980s (MacCoun and Reuter, 1997). Between 1984 and 1996 the use of cannabis in Holland increased rapidly, with lifetime exposure in the 18- to 20-year-old group rising from 15% in 1984 to 44% in 1996, and previous month exposure rising from 8.5% to 18.5%. However, similar rapid increases in cannabis consumption in this age group were observed during the 1990s in the United States and in Norway, two countries that have strictly enforced prohibition laws. There is some evidence that the Dutch consumption of cannabis rose faster during the 1980s than elsewhere, probably as a result of the coffee shop policy. The fact remains that the current levels of cannabis use among young people in Holland are comparable to those in other European countries and considerably lower than those in the United States, even after 30 years of decriminalization. Reinarman et al. (2004) surveyed groups of cannabis users in Amsterdam and San Francisco:

> We compared representative samples of experienced marijuana users to see whether the lawful availability of marijuana did, in fact, lead to the problems critics of the Dutch system have claimed. We found no evidence that it does. In fact, we found consistently strong similarities in patterns of marijuana use, despite vastly different national drug policies.

Among their findings were that the age of onset of cannabis use and the age at which regular use commenced was very similar in the two cities; 75% in each city used cannabis less than once a week and there was little evidence in either city that cannabis was a gateway drug to other more dangerous narcotics, although users in San Francisco were more likely to proceed to cocaine, amphetamines, or opiates than those in Holland. Whether the Dutch experiment has succeeded in its objective of separating the use of soft and hard drugs is not easy to prove. There are some positive data: for example, the average age of heroin addicts in Holland is increasing—suggesting that fewer young people are being recruited to heroin addiction. In 1981, 14% of Dutch heroin addicts were under 22; today that figure is less than 5%. In 1995 the number of heroin addicts per 100,000 population was 160 in Holland versus 430 per 100,000 in the United States. But there remains an association between cannabis use and exposure to other psychoactive drugs—cannabis users are far more likely to have experimented with other psychoactive drugs than nondrug users. It is perhaps too early to say how successful the experiment has been in this regard (Ossebaard, 1996). The Dutch approach would not fit easily in many other countries. It requires an ability to "look the other way," which others might find more difficult. The coffee shop customers come through the front door and purchase small amounts of cannabis with impunity, but the coffee shop owners have no legal source of supply. They must obtain supplies of cannabis where they can, and have them delivered through the back door. More than half of all cannabis consumed in Holland is home grown—with increasing horticultural expertise and new strains of high THC content cannabis plants. The rest is imported, mainly from Morocco. But the suppliers are still liable to criminal penalties if caught. Other European countries have complained that Holland has become an easy source of supply of cannabis for drug tourists from all over Europe who may carry away their purchases with little risk across a European Union that no longer has many border controls. Public opinion in Holland is by no means unanimously in favor of the present relaxed drug laws. Increased tightening of the regulations has led to the closure of hundreds of coffee shops, and there have been moves to limit the sale of cannabis to Dutch nationals only. A parliamentary move to provide legal sources of supply for coffee shops was recently blocked by the conservative government.

The Dutch experiment has not been repeated anywhere else so far, although some states in the United States decriminalized cannabis possession for a while in the 1970s, and there have been moves toward this in California and elsewhere more recently. As in the Netherlands, this did not seem to lead to any marked increase in cannabis consumption (Institute of Medicine, 1999). The possession of small amounts of cannabis for personal use is also no longer punished in Belgium, Spain, or Italy, or in some states in Australia. The country that seemed most likely to follow the Dutch in permitting the sale of cannabis from licensed premises was Switzerland, where the government has tried four times since 2001 to introduce a law that would permit the supply and sale of small quantities of cannabis, but parliament has voted against the legislation on each occasion, most recently in 2004. France and Germany remain firmly attached to their present policies of prohibition and punishment.

Meanwhile, however, Britain has experienced a sudden relaxation of the cannabis laws in the past few years. Throughout the 1990s British public opinion about cannabis became increasingly tolerant (Warburton et al., 2005). In 2000 the results of an Independent Inquiry into the Misuse of Drugs Act 1971, undertaken by the Police Foundation and chaired by Dame Ruth Runciman, was published. The review panel had included senior policemen and a variety of scientific, medical, and legal experts. Its conclusions were radical and clearcut, and some have been reviewed in previous chapters. One of the recommendations of the Runciman report was that cannabis should no longer be a Class B substance under the Misuse of Drugs Act 1971, but should be downgraded. The review went on to state:

> We have encountered a wide sense of unease, indeed scepticism, about the present control regime in respect of cannabis. It inhibits accurate education about the relative risks of different drugs, including cannabis itself. It gives large numbers of otherwise law-abiding people a criminal record. It inordinately penalises and marginalises young people for what might be little more than youthful experimentation. It bears most heavily on young people on the streets of inner cities, who are also more likely to be poor and members of minority ethnic groups. The evidence strongly indicates that the current law and its operation create more harm than the drug itself.

At almost the same time, the opposition Conservative party Shadow Home Secretary Ann Widdicombe proposed exactly the opposite sort of policy when she addressed the Conservative Party Conference in October 2000. She demanded a zero tolerance attitude toward cannabis possession and use, with mandatory minimum fines of £100 for possession. Her gambit backfired spectacularly; within a few days five of her colleagues in the Shadow cabinet had broken ranks, admitting that they themselves had at one time used cannabis. Meanwhile, the newspapers, which usually denounced politicians as being too liberal on drug policy, lampooned her for being out of touch!

The British government rejected the recommendations of the Runciman report shortly after its publication, but various senior police officers advocated reform, and an experimental scheme was launched in the Lambeth district of London in which police officers delivered on-the-spot warnings instead of arrests to those found in possession of cannabis. In 2001 the newly appointed Home Secretary, David Blunkett, announced his intention to consider downgrading cannabis. The Home Office Advisory Council on the Misuse of Drugs (ACMD) undertook a thorough independent review and recommended that cannabis be downgraded from Class B to C—which duly took effect in January 2004. In fact, the police in many parts of Britain had already been treating cannabis offenders more leniently for several years before this change took place (Warburton et al., 2005).

This was not the end of the story, however, as some newspapers and British politicians continued to argue against this liberalization of the cannabis laws, and influential figures in the field of academic psychiatry warned of new reports linking teenage cannabis use to subsequent mental illness (see Chapter 6), while others warned of the possible health risks of high potency "skunk" (see Chapter 7). David Blunkett's successor as Home Secretary, Charles Clarke, asked the Home Office ACMD to look again at this new evidence and to recommend whether cannabis should again be reclassified into Class B. After careful deliberation the Committee recommended against this, stating:

> Cannabis is harmful and its consumption can lead to a wide range of physical and psychological hazards. Nevertheless the Council does not advise that the classification of cannabis-containing products should be changed on the basis of the results of recent research into the effects on the development of mental illness. Although it is unquestionably harmful, its harmfulness does not equate to that of other Class B substances either at the level of the individual or of society." (Advisory Council on the Misuse of Drugs, 2005)

While European countries are tending to view illegal drug use as a public health problem, the United States continues to wage war on drugs with the full force of the criminal law.

Marijuana arrests reached an all-time high of 786,545 in 2005, having more than doubled since 1992 (Fig. 8.1). A majority (88%) of arrests

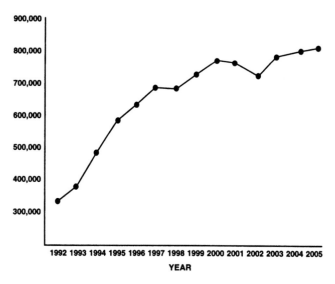

**Figure 8.1.** Marijuana arrests in the United States. (Data from http://normal.
org/index.cfm?Group_ID=7040)

were for simple possession. Marijuana continues to be viewed as America's
number one drug problem by the Drug Enforcement Agency, who consistently criticize the Dutch experiment and emphasize the dangers of marijuana use. Punishments vary widely across the country, from modest fines
to a few days to many years in prison. Alabama currently locks up people
convicted three times of marijuana *possession* for 15 years to life. More
than 60,000 nonviolent cannabis offenders are in American prisons, often
with long sentences. A parent's marijuana use can be the basis for taking away his or her children and putting them in foster care. Foreign-born
residents of the United States can be deported for a marijuana offense, no
matter low long they have been legally employed. More than half the states
revoke or suspend driver's licenses of people arrested for marijuana possession, even though they were not driving at the time of the arrest. This is
clearly overreaction by any standards.

The White House Office of National Drug Control Policy (ONDCP) continues to campaign against marijuana and to encourage random drug testing in schools and colleges. An anti-marijuana advertising campaign aimed at teenagers has cost more than $2 billion since 1998 and continues, despite little evidence of its effectiveness. But although the federal government has adhered strictly to its anti-cannabis policies, an uncomfortable dichotomy has developed between it and the opinions of voters in several parts of the United States. As described previously, the use of marijuana for medical purposes has been approved by voters in 12 states, and the practice of providing medical marijuana continues, although the federal government continues to attempt to stop it. The government scored a victory in a Supreme Court ruling in 2005, giving the federal government the power to arrest and prosecute patients and their suppliers even if the marijuana use is permitted under state law. Patients are increasingly worried about their personal risk of arrest, and marijuana pharmacies are raided regularly by federal agents (Okie, 2005). On the day that the Supreme Court ruling was announced, John Walters, the U.S. drug czar said:

> Today's decision marks the end of medical marijuana as a political issue.... We have a responsibility as a civilized society to ensure that the medicine Americans receive from their doctors is effective, safe, and free from the pro-drug politics that are being promoted in America under the guise of medicine. (Okie, 2005)

However, there have been few federally sponsored patient arrests and the long-running battle between federal state governments over the medical use of marijuana is far from over.

## What Next? Is There a Case for the Legalization/ Decriminalization/Depenalization of Cannabis?

Although unthinkable only a few years ago, a debate has begun on both sides of the Atlantic about the possibility of removing cannabis from its current criminal status. In the United States, influential figures from both major political parties have joined this debate, and opinion polls have shown a majority in favor of the proposition that for simple marijuana possession, people should not be incarcerated but fined, the generally accepted definition of *decriminalization* (Nadelmann, 2004). As Nadelmann put it:

> Marijuana prohibition is unique among American criminal laws. No other law is both enforced so widely and harshly and yet deemed unnecessary by such a substantial portion of the populace.

There have been moves at a local level in the United States to reduce the penalties associated with possession of small amounts of cannabis for personal use. In the November 2006 elections voters in Nevada and Colorado were asked to approve such decriminalization of cannabis. Although the propositions were not approved, 40% of voters in Colorado and 44% in Nevada voted in favor, and some local municipalities in these and other states did approve similar measures.

In Britain such sober newspapers as the *Daily Telegraph*, *The Independent*, and *The Economist* have published editorials in favor of the outright legalization or decriminalization of cannabis, as has the editor of the medical journal *The Lancet*:

> The smoking of cannabis, even long term, is not harmful to health. (*Lancet*, Nov. 11, 1995)

In 2001 Peter Lilley, a former deputy leader of the Conservative Party, published a pamphlet in Britain calling for the legalization of cannabis, recommending that it be made available for sale under license with a ban on sales to those under 18. He recommended that cannabis sales be taxed and that growing it for personal use should be allowed.

Apart from the Netherlands the country that has gone furthest down the path to decriminalization is Australia, where some state governments decided to adopt some form of *depenalization*—that is, to remove penal sanctions for cannabis possession (and in some cases cultivation) for personal use. Wayne Hall (2007) reviewed the Australian experience and summarized what he calls "a cautious case for cannabis depenalization." Some of the arguments are worth listing here. Having reviewed the various health hazards associated with cannabis use (see Chapter 5), he discusses the "arguments for cannabis liberalization." These include (1) the libertarian argument—that individuals should be able to decide for themselves whether to enjoy the pleasurable effects of cannabis; (2) the hypocrisy of allowing alcohol to be sold legally while keep cannabis illegal—when the two drugs are of comparable harmfulness; (3) the social and economic costs of cannabis prohibition outweighing the benefits; and (4) that prohibition has failed to deter young people from using cannabis. He goes on to list the "social costs of prohibition." These include (1) the large monetary costs of enforcing the cannabis laws—including costs to the police, court system, and prisons; (2) the costs of the black market—which artificially raises the cost of cannabis to compensate for the risks of arrest and punishment incurred by the illegal sellers; (3) the potential for corruption of law enforcement officials because of the huge profits made in the black market; (4) the lack of any regulation of the quality of cannabis sold on the black market; (5) the potential tax revenues that are forgone; (6) the fact that the system imposes a penalty that is disproportionate to any harm caused by the offense; and (7) the fact that education suffers as governments tend to give misleading information about the health effects of cannabis in order to justify their policies, and as a result young people are sceptical about *all* information on the adverse effects of the drug. Hall, in what he describes as a "choice of evils," comes down in favor of a policy of depenalization, although this has the major weakness of failing to address the problems created by a black market for the supply of illegal cannabis, and it cannot be viewed as a long-term solution.

These ideas go a long way further than the downgrading from Class B to C that took place in Britain in 2004. Cannabis remains an illegal drug in Britain, and the penalties for dealing were made even harsher as a political sweetener to opponents of the downgrading. One lesson that the downgrading exercise in Britain has reinforced is that, as in the Netherlands, changes in the law have had little effect on cannabis consumption. Critics had predicted that downgrading would lead to an explosion in cannabis use, but the statistics actually show a continuing decline in use by young people—a trend that has been going on ever since the year 2000 (Table 7.6).

It is hard to predict where changes in the laws governing cannabis will go in the future. Sometimes large changes in social policy and human behavior take place very quickly—as in the reform of the laws governing divorce or those on homosexuality, or the banning of tobacco smoking in public places. Whether such sudden shifts will happen in the case of cannabis is still unclear—but the pace of change toward a grudging acceptance of cannabis as part of modern life may ultimately prove irresistible.

Politicians, ever mindful that the cannabis debate remains highly polarized, are likely to continue to suffer from the syndrome described below:

> Cannabis can cause anxiety, agitation, and anger among politicians. The consequences of this cannabis-induced psychological distress syndrome (CIPDS) include over-reaction with respects to legislation and politics and a lack of distinction between use and misuse of cannabis. (*Lancet*, May 15th, 2004)

# References

Abel EL. *Marihuana. The First Twelve Thousand Years.* New York: Plenum Press; 1943 (reprinted 1980).

Abood ME. Molecular biology of cannabinoid receptors. *Handb Exp Pharmacol.* 2005;168:81–116.

Abood ME and Martin BR. Neurobiology of marijuana abuse. *Trends Pharmacol Science.* 2002;13:201–206.

Abrams DI, Jay CA, Vizoso H, et al. Cannabis in HIV-associated sensory neuropathy. *Neurology.* 2005;68:515–521.

Adams IB, Martin BR. Cannabis: pharmacology and toxicology in animals and humans. *Addiction.* 1996;91:1585–1614.

Adams R. Marihuana. *Harvey Lect.* 1941–1942;37:168–197.

Advisory Committee on Drug Dependence. *Cannabis.* London: Her Majesty's Stationery Office; 1969.

Advisory Council on the Misuse of Drugs. *Further Consideration of Classification of Cannabis under the Misuse of Drugs Act 1971.* London: Home Office; 2005.

Advisory Council on the Misuse of Drugs. *Pathways to Problems.* London: Home Office; 2006.

Agurell S, Halldin M, Lindgren J-E, et al. Pharmacokinetics and metabolism of $\Delta^1$-tetrahydrocannabinol and other cannabinoids with emphasis on man. *Pharmacol Rev.* 1986;38:21–38.

Alger BA. Endocannabinoids: getting the message across. *Proc Nat Acad Sci USA.* 2004;101:8512–8513.

American Medical Association. *Report of the Council on Scientific Affairs to AMA House of Delegates on Medical Marijuana.* CSA Report I-97; 1997.

American Psychiatric Association. *Diagnostic and Statistical Manual of Mental Disorders (DSM-IV).* 4th ed. Washington D.C.: American Psychiatric Association; 1994.

Andreasson S, Allebeck P, Engstrom A, Rydberg U. Cannabis and schizophrenia. A longitudinal study of Swedish conscripts. *Lancet*. 1987;ii:1483–1485.

Andreasson S, Allebeck P, Rydberg U. Schizophrenia in users and nonusers of cannabis. *Acta Psychiatr Scand*. 1989;79:505–510.

Anslinger H, Cooper CR. Marihuana: assassin of youth. *American Magazine*. 1937;July:150.

Arevola-Martin A, Vela JM, Molina-Holgado E, Borrell J, Guaza C. Therapeutic action of cannabinoids in a murine model of multiple sclerosis. *J Neurosci*. 2003;23:2511–2516.

Armentano P. Emerging clinical applications for cannabis and cannabinoids. A review of the recent scientific literature, 2000–2006. National Organization for the Reform of Marijuana Laws. Available at: http://www.norml.org; 2006.

Arseneault L, Cannon M, Witton J, Murray RM. Causal association between cannabis and psychosis: examination of the evidence. *Br J Psychiatry*. 2004;184:110–117.

Atha MJ. Cannabinoids and multiple sclerosis. Independent Drug Monitoring Unit. Available at: http://www.idmu.co.uk/canmsreview.htm; 2005.

Axelrod J, Felder C. Cannabinoid receptors and their endogenous agonist anandamide. *Neurochemical Res*. 1998;23:575–581.

Baddeley A. The fractionation of working memory. *Proc Natl Acad Sci USA*. 1996;93:13468–13472.

Baker D, Pryce G, Croxford JL, et al. Endocannabinoids control spasticity in a multiple sclerosis model. *FASEB J*. 2001;15:300–302.

Baker D, Pryce G, Davies WL, Hiley CR. In silico patent searching reveals a new cannabinoid receptor. *Trends Pharmacol Sci*. 2006;27:1–4.

Bari M, Battista N, Gezza F, et al. New insights into endocannabinoid degradation and its therapeutic potential. *Mini Rev Med Chem*. 2006;6:257–268.

Barnes MP. Sativex: clinical efficacy and tolerability in the treatment of symptoms of multiple sclerosis and neuropathic pain. *Expert Opin Pharmacother*. 2006;7:607–615.

Beal JE, et al. Dronabinol as a treatment for anorexia associated with weight loss in patients with AIDS. *J Pain Symptom Manage*. 1995;10:89–97.

Bédard M, Dubois S, Weaver B. The impact of cannabis on driving. *Can J Public Health*. 2007;98:6–11.

Bell R, Wechsler H, Johnston LD. Correlates of college student marijuana use: results of a US National Survey. *Addiction*. 1997;92:571–581.

Bellochio L, Mancini G, Vicennati V, et al. Cannabinoid receptors as therapeutic targets for obesity and metabolic diseases. *Curr Opin Pharmacol*. 2006;6:586–591.

Beltramo M, Stella N, Calignano A, et al. Functional role of high-affinity anandamide transport, as revealed by selective inhibition. *Science*. 1997;277:1094–1097.

Berke J, Hernton C. *The Cannabis Experience*. Aylesbury, UK: Hazell Watson & Viney. London: Quartet Books Ltd; 1974 (reprinted 1977).

Berman JS, Symonds C, Birch R. Efficacy of two cannabis based medicinal extracts for relief of central neuropathic pain from brachial plexus avulsion: results of a randomised controlled trial. *Pain*. 2004;112:299–306.

Bertolini A, Ferrari A, Ottani A, et al. Paracetamol: new vista of an old drug. *CNS Drug Rev*. 2006;12:250–275.

Bisogno T, Cascio MG, Saha B, et al. Development of the first potent and specific inhibitors of endocannabinoid biosynthesis. *Biochim Biophys Acta*. 2006;1761:205–212.

Blake DR, Robson P, Ho M, et al. Preliminary assessment of the efficacy, tolerability and safety of a cannabis-based medicine (Sativex) in the treatment of pain caused by rheumatoid arthritis. *Rheumatology*. 2006;45:50–52.

Block RI, O'Leary DS, Ehrhardt JC, et al. Effects of frequent marijuana use on brain tissue volume and composition. *Neuroreport*. 2000;11:491–496.

Bonnie RJ, Whitbread CH. *The Marihuana Conviction. A History of Marihuana Prohibition in the Unites States*. Charlottesville, VA: University Press of Virginia; 1974.

Booth M. *Cannabis: A History*. London: Transworld Publishers; 2003.

Bortolato M, Campolongo P, Mangieri RA, et al. Anxiolytic-like properties of the anandamide transport inhibitor AM404. *Neuropsychopharmacology*. 2006;31:2652–2659.

Bowman M and Pihl RO. Cannabis: psychological effects of chronic heavy use. A controlled study of intellectual functioning in chronic users of high potency. *Psychopharmacologia*. 1973;29:159–170.

Brady CM, DasGupta R, Dalton C, et al. An open-label pilot study of cannabis-based extracts for bladder dysfunction in advanced multiple sclerosis. *Mult Scler*. 2004;10:425–433.

Braude MC. Toxicology of cannabinoids. In: Paton WM, Crown J (eds). *Cannabis and Its Derivatives*. Oxford: Oxford University Press; 1972:89–99.

British Medical Association. *Therapeutic Uses of Cannabis*. UK Harwood Academic Publishers Amsterdam; 1997.

Budney AJ, Hughes JR, Moore BA, Novy PL. Marijuana abstinence effects in marijuana smokers maintained in their home environment. *Arch Gen Psychiatry*. 2001;58:917–924.

Cabral GA, Staab A. Effects on the immune system. *Handb Exp Pharmacol*. 2005;168:386–423.

Campbell FA, Tramer MR, Carroll D, et al. Are cannabinoids an effective and safe treatment option in the management of pain? A qualitative systematic review. *BMJ*, 2001;323:13–16.

Canadian Government Commission of Inquiry into the Non-Medical Use of Drugs. *Cannabis*. Ottawa: Information Canada; 1970.

Carai M, Colombo G, Maccioni P, Gessa GL. Efficacy of rimonabant and other cannabinoid CB-1 receptor antagonists in reducing food intake and body weight: preclinical and clinical data. *CNS Drug Rev.* 2006;12:91–99.

Caspi A, Moffitt TE, Cannon M, et al. Moderation of the effect of adolescent-onset cannabis use on adult psychosis by a functional polymorphism in the catechol-O-methyl transferase gene: longitudinal evidence of a gene X environment interaction. *Biol Psychiatry.* 2005;57:1117–1127.

Castle DJ, Murray R, (eds). *Marijuana and Madness.* Cambridge: Cambridge University Press; 2004.

Centonze D, Finazzi-Agro A, Bernardi G, Maccarrone M. The endocannabinoid system in targeting inflammatory neurodegenerative diseases. *Trends Pharmacol Sci.* 2007;28:180–187.

Chan GCK, Hinds TR, Impey S, Storm DR. Hippocampal neurotoxicity of Δ9-tetrahydrocannabinol. *J Neurosci.* 1998;18:5322–5332.

Chan PC, Sills RC, Braun AG, Haseman JK, Bucher JR. Toxicity and carcinogenicity of delta-9-tetrahydrocannabinol in Fischer rats and B6C3F1 mice. *Fundament Appl Toxicol.* 1996;30:109–117.

Chopra IC, Chopra RN. The use of cannabis drugs in India. *Bull Narc.* 1957;Jan:4–29.

Clarke RC. *Marijuana Botany.* Berkeley, CA: Ronin Publishing; 1981.

Comitas L. Cannabis and work in Jamaica: a refutation of the amotivational syndrome. *Ann NY Acad Sci.* 1976;282:24–32.

Consroe PF, Snider R. Therapeutic potential of cannabinoids in neurological disorders. In: Mechoulam R (ed). *Cannabinoids as Therapeutic Agents.* Boca Raton, FL: CRC Press; 1986:21–49.

Costa B, Sinicalco D, Trovata AE, et al. AM404, an inhibitor of anandamide uptake, prevents pain behaviour and modulates cytokine and apoptotic pathways in a rat model of neuropathic pain. *Br J Pharmacol.* 2006;148:1022–1032.

Cravatt BF, Giang DK, Mayfield SP, et al. Molecular characterization of an enzyme that degrades neuromodulatory fatty acid amides. *Nature.* 1996;384:83–87.

Cravatt BF, Demarest K, Patricelli MP, et al. Supersensitivity to anandamide and enhanced endocannabinoid signaling in mice lacking fatty acid amide hydrolase. *Proc Nat Acad Sci USA.* 2001;98:9371–9376.

D'Ambra TE, et al. C-attached aminoalkylindoles: potent cannabinoid mimetics. *Bioorganic Med Chem Lett.* 1996;6:17–22.

De Fonseca FR, Carrera MRA, Navarro M, Koob GF, Weiss F. Activation of corticotropin-releasing factor in the limbic system during cannabinoid withdrawal. *Science.* 1997;276:2050–2054.

Degenhardt L, Hall W, Lynskey M. Testing hypotheses about the relationship between cannabis use and psychosis. *Drug Alcohol Depend.* 2003;71:37–48.

Denton TF, Earleywine M. Pothead or pot smoker? A taxometric investigation of cannabis dependence. *Subst Abuse Treat Prev Policy.* 2006;1:22.

Devane WA, Dysarz A, Johnson MR, Melvin LS, Howlett A. Determination and characterization of a cannabinoid receptor in rat brain. *Mol Pharmacol.* 1988;34:605–613.

Devane WA, Hanus L, Breuer A, et al. Isolation and structure of a brain constituent that binds to the cannabinoid receptor. *Science.* 1992;258:1946–1949.

Dickson-Chesterfield AK, Kidd SR, Moore SA, et al. Pharmacological characterization of endocannabinoid transport and fatty acid amide hydrolase inhibitors. *Cell Mol Neurobiol.* 2006;26:405–421.

Di Marzo V, De Petrocellis L, Bisogno T. The biosynthesis, fate and pharmacological properties of endocannabinoids. *Handb Exp Pharmacol.* 2005;168:147–185.

Dixon WE. The pharmacology of cannabis indica. *BMJ.* 1899;Nov 11:1354–1357.

Doll R, Peto R, Boreham J, Sutherland I. Mortality from cancer in relation to smoking: 50 years observations on British doctors. *Br J Cancer.* 2005;92:426–429.

Downer EJ, Boland B, Fogarty M, Campbell V. Δ⁹-Tetrahydrocannabinol induces the apoptotic pathway in cultured cortical neurones via activation of the $CB_1$ receptor. *NeuroReport.* 2001;12:3973–3978.

D'Souza DC, Perry E, MacDougall L, et al. The psychotomimetic effects of intravenous delta-9-tetrahydrocannabinol in healthy individuals: implications for psychosis. *Neuropsychopharmacology.* 2004;29:1558–1572.

Duane Sofia R. Cannabis: structure-activity relationships. In: Iversen LL, Iversen SD, Snyder SH (eds). *Handbook of Psychopharmacology.* Vol. 12. New York: Plenum Press; 1978:319–371.

Earleywine M. *Understanding Marijuana.* Oxford: Oxford University Press; 2002.

El Sohly MA. Suppository formulations effecting bioavailability of delta-9-THC. US Patent 5,508,03, issued April 16, 1996 (divisional application of US Patent 5,389,375).

Egertová M, Elphick MR. Localisation of cannabinoid receptors in the rat brain using antibodies to the intracellular C-terminal tail of $CB_1$. *J Comp Neurol.* 2000;422:159–171.

Egertová M, Giang DK, Cravatt BF, Elphick MR. A new perspective on cannabinoid signalling: complementary localisation of fatty acid amide hydrolase and the CB1 receptor in rat brain. *Proc R Soc Lond B Biol Sci.* 1998;265:2081–2085.

Elphick MR, Egertová M. The neurobiology and evolution of cannabinoid signaling. *Phil Trans R Soc Lond.* 2001;356:381–408.

Emrich HM, Leweke FM, Schneider U. Towards a cannabinoid hypothesis of schizophrenia: cognitive impairments due to dysregulation of the endogenous cannabinoid system. *Pharmacol Biochem Behav.* 1997;56:8030–8080.

Engelsman EL. Dutch policy on the management of drug-related problems. *Br J Addict,* 1989;84:211–218.

Fegley D, Kathuria S, Mercier R, et al. Anandamide transport is independent of fatty acid amide hydrolase activity and is blocked by the hydrolysis-resistant inhibitor AM1172. *Proc Nat Acad Sci USA.* 2004;101:8756–8761.

Felder CC, Glass M. Cannabinoid receptors and their endogenous agonists. *Ann Rev Pharmacol Toxicol.* 1998;38:179–200.

Fergusson DM, Horwood LJ, Ridder EM. Tests of causal linkage between cannabis use and psychotic symptoms. *Addiction.* 2005;100:354–366.

Fernández-Ruiz J, González S. Cannabinoid control of motor function at the basal ganglia. *Handb Exp Pharmacol.* 2005;168:479–508.

Fields HL, Meng ID. Watching the pot boil: selective antagonists of the two cannabinoid receptors unveil distinct but synergistic peripheral analgesic activities for endogenous cannabinoids. *Nat Med.* 1998;4:1000–1009.

Fletcher JM, Page JB, Francis DJ, et al. Cognitive correlates of long-term cannabis use in Costa Rican men. *Arch Gen Psychiatry.* 1996;53:1051–1057.

Freeman RM, Adekanmi O, Waterfield MR, et al. The effect of cannabis on urge incontinence in patients with multiple sclerosis: a multicentre, randomised placebo-controlled trial (CAMS-LUTS). *Int Urognynecol J Pelvic Floor Dysfunct.* 2006;17:636–641.

French ED, Dillon K, Wu X. Cannabinoids excite dopamine neurons in the ventral tegmentum and substantia nigra. *NeuroReport.* 1997;8:649–652.

Fried PA. Prenatal exposure to tobacco and marijuana: effects during pregnancy, infancy, and early childhood. *Clin Obstet Gynecol.* 1993;36:319–337.

Fried PA, Watkinson B, Gray R. Differential effects on cognitive functioning in 13- to 16-year-olds prenatally exposed to cigarettes and marihuana. *Neurotoxicol Teratol.* 2003;25:427–436.

Fries JF. Assessing and understanding patient risk. *Scand J Rheumatol.* 1992;92(Suppl):21–24.

Gettman G. Marijuana production in the United States (2006). *Bull Cannabis Reform.* 2006;December.

Ghodse H. When too much caution can be harmful. *Addiction.* 1996;91:764–766.

Gieringer D, St Laurent J, Goodrich S. Cannabis vaporiser combines efficient delivery of THC without effecting supply of pyrolytic compounds. *J Cannabis Ther.* 2004;4:7–27.

Giuffrida A, Parsons LH, Kerr TM, de Fonseca FR, Navarro M, Piomelli D. Dopamine activation of endogenous cannabinoid signalling in dorsal striatum. *Nat Neurosci.* 1999;2:358–363.

Goode E. *The Marijuana Smokers.* New York: Basic Books Inc; 1970.

Gorter RW, Butorac M, Cobian EP, van der Sluis W. Medical use of cannabis in the Netherlands. *Neurology.* 2005;64:917–919.

Grinspoon L, Bakalar JB. *Marihuana, the Forbidden Medicine.* New Haven, CT: Yale University Press; 1993 (revised 1997).

Guzman M. Effects on cell viability. *Handb Exp Pharmacol.* 2005;168:627–642.

Guzman M, Duarte MJ, Blazquez C, et al. A pilot clinical study of Delta-9-terahydrocannabinol in patients with recurrent glioblastoma. *Br J Cancer.* 2006;95:197–203.

Hall W. A cautious case for cannabis depenalization. In: Earleywine M (ed). *Pot Politics.* Oxford: Oxford University Press; 2007:91–112.

Hall W, Solowij N. Long-term cannabis use and mental health. *Br J Psychiatry.* 1997;171:107–108.

Hall W, Solowij N, Lemon J. The Health and Psychological Consequences of Cannabis Use. Monograph Series No 25, National Drug Strategy. Canberra: Australian Government Publishing Service; 1994.

Han CJ, Robinson JK. Cannabinoid modulation of time estimation in the rat. *Behav Neurosci.* 2001;115:243–246.

Harper JW, Heath RG, Myers WA. Effects of cannabis sativa on ultrastructure of the synapse in monkey brain. *J Neurosci Res.* 1977;3:87–93.

Hashibe M, Morgenstern H, Cui Y, et al. Marijuana use and the risk of lung and upper aerodigestive tract cancers: results of a population based case-control study. *Cancer Epidemiol Biomarkers Prev.* 2006;15:1829–1834.

Hashibe M, Straif K, Tashkin DP, et al. Epidemiologic review of marijuana use and cancer risk. *Alcohol.* 2005;35:265–275.

Heath RG, Fitzjarrel AT, Fontana CJ, Garey RE. Cannabis sativa: effects on brain function and ultrastructure in rhesus monkeys. *Biol Psychiatry.* 1980;15:657–691.

Heishman SJ, Stitzer M, Yinglilng JE. Effects of tetrahydrocannabinol content on marijuana smoking behaviour, subjective reports, and performance. *Pharmacol Biochem Behav.* 1989;34:173–179.

Henquet C, Murray R, Linszen D, van Os J. The environment and schizophrenia: the role of cannabis use. *Schizophrenia Bull.* 2005;31:608–612.

Herkenham M, Lynn AB, Johnson MR, Melvin LS, de Costa BR, Rice KC. Characterization and localization of cannabinoid receptors in rat brain: a quantitative *in vitro* autoradiographic study. *J Neurosci.* 1991;11:563–583.

Herning RI, Hooker WT, Jones RT. Tetrahydrocannabinol content and differences in marijuana smoking behaviour. *Psychopharmacology.* 1986;90:160–162.

Hickman M, Vickerman P, Macleod J, Kirkbride J, Jones PB. Cannabis and schizophrenia: model projections of the impact of the rise in cannabis use on historical and future trends in schizophrenia in England and Wales. *Addiction.* 2007;102:597–606.

Himmelstein JL. The strange career of marihuana. *Contributions in Political Science,* No 94. Westport, CT: Greenwood Press; 1978.

Ho WSV, Hillard CJ. Modulators of endocannabinoid enzyme hydrolysis and membrane transport. *Handb Exp Pharmacol.* 2005;168:188–207.

Högestatt ED, Jönsson BAG, Ermund A, et al. Conversion of acetaminophen to the bioactive N-acylphenolamine AM404 via fatty acid amide hydrolase-dependent arachidonic acid conjugation in the nervous system. *J Biol Chem.* 2005;280:31405–31412.

Hohmann AG, Suplita RL, Bolton NM, et al. An endocannabinoid mechanism for stress-induced analgesia. *Nature.* 2005;435:1108–1111.

Hollister LE. Health Aspects of Cannabis. *Pharmacol Rev.* 1986;38:1–20.

Hollister LE. Health aspects of cannabis: revisited. *Int J Neuropsychopharmacol.* 1998;1:71–80.

Horti AG, Fan H, Kuwabara H, et al. 11C-JHU75528: a radiotracer for PET imaging of CB1 cannabinoid receptors. *J Nucl Med.* 2006;47:1689–1696.

House of Lords, Select Committee on Science and Technology. Cannabis—The Scientific and Medical Evidence. London: The Stationery Office; 1998.

Howlett AC. Cannabinoid receptor signalling. *Handb Exp Pharmacol.* 2005; 168:53–80.

Huestis MA. Pharmacokinetics and metabolism of the plant cannabinoids, Δ⁹-tetrahydrocannabinol, cannabidiol and cannabinol. *Handb Exp Pharmacol.* 2005;168:657–690.

Huestis MA, Gorelick DA, Heishman SJ, et al. Blockade of effects of smoked marijuana by the CB1-selective cannabinoid receptor antagonist SR141716. *Arch Gen Psychiatry.* 2001;58:322–328.

Huestis MA, Sampson AH, Holicky BJ, Henningfield JE, Cone EJ. Characterization of the absorption phase of marijuana smoking. *Clin Pharmacol Ther.* 1992;52:31–41.

Indian Hemp Drugs Commission. Report. Simla, India: Government Central Printing Office; 1894.

Institute of Medicine. Joy JE, Watson Jr J, Benson Jr JA (eds). *Marijuana and Medicine.* Washington DC: National Academy Press; 1999.

Iversen LL. Cannabis and the brain. *Brain.* 2003;126:1252–1260.

Iversen LL, Chapman V. Cannabinoids: a real prospect for pain relief? *Curr Opin Pharmacol.* 2002;2:50–55.

Izzo AA, Capasso F. Marijuana for cholera therapy. *Trends Pharmac Sci.* 2006; 27:7–8.

Jahr GHG. *New Homeopathic Pharmacopoeia and Posology or the Preparation of Homeopathic Medicines.* Philadelphia: J. Dobson; 1842:137.

Johns A. Psychiatric effects of cannabis. *Br J Psychiatry.* 2001;178:116–122.

Johnson JR, GWCA101 Investigator Group, Potts RL. *Cannabis-Based Medicines in the Treatment of Cancer Pain—Preliminary Results* [Abstract]. Sydney: IASP; August 21–26, 2005.

Kandel DB, Davies M. High school students who use crack and other drugs. *Arch Gen Psychiatry.* 1996;53:71–80.

Kaslow RA, Blackwelder WC, Ostrow DG, et al. No evidence for a role of alcohol or other psychoactive drugs in accelerating immunodeficiency in HIV-1-positive individuals. *JAMA.* 1989;261:3424–3429.

Katona I, Sperlagh B, Sik A, et al. Presynaptically located $CB_1$ receptors regulate GABA release from axon terminals of specific hippocampal interneurons. *J Neurosci.* 1999;19:4544–4558.

King LA, Carpenties C, Griffiths P. An Overview of Cannabis Potency in Europe. European Monitoring Centre for Drugs and Drug Abuse; 2004.

Kolodny RC, Masters WH, Kolodner RM, Toro G. Depression of plasma testosterone levels after chronic intensive marihuana use. *New Engl J Med.* 1974;290:872–874.

Korf DJ, Wouter M, Benschop A, van Ginkel P. *Sterke Wiet.* Amsterdam: Rozenburg Publishers; 2004.

Kozlowski LT, Wilkinson DA, Skinner W, et al. Comparing tobacco cigarette dependence with other drug dependencies. *JAMA.* 1989;261:898–901.

Kuster JE, Stevenson JI, Ward SJ, D'Ambra TE, Haycock DA. Aminoalkylindole binding in rat cerebellum: selective displacement by natural and synthetic cannabinoids. *J Pharmacol Exp Ther.* 1993;264:1352–1363.

Lambert DM, Fowler CJ. The endocannabinoid system: drug targets, lead compounds, and potential therapeutic applications. *J Med Chem.* 2005;48:5059–5087.

Ledent C, et al. Unresponsiveness to cannabinoids and reduced addictive effects of opiates in $CB_1$ receptor knockout mice. *Science.* 1999;283:401.

Lemberger L. Clinical evaluation of cannabinoids in the treatment of disease. In: Harvey DJ, Paton W, Nahas G (eds). *Marihuana '84.* Oxford: IRL Press Ltd; 1985:673–680.

Levine JD, Gordon NC, Bornstein JC, Fields HL. Role of pain in placebo analgesia. *Proc Natl Acad Sci USA.* 1979;76:3528–3531.

Levitt M, Faiman C, Hawks R, Wilson A. Randomized double-blind comparison of delta-9-tetrahydrocannabinol (THC) and marijuana as chemotherapy antiemetics. *Proc Amer Soc Clin Oncol.* 1984;3:91.

Lewin L. PHANTASTICA. *Narcotic and Stimulating Drugs their Use and Abuse.* London: Routledge & Kegan Paul; 1931.

Lichtman AH, Martin BR. Cannabinoid tolerance and dependence. *Handb Exp Pharmacol.* 2005;168:691–717.

Ligresti A, Moriello AS, Starowicz K, et al. Antitumor activity of plant cannabinoids with emphasis on the effect of cannabidiol on human breast carcinoma. *J Pharmacol Exp Ther.* 2006;318:1375–1387.

Lindsey KP, Glaser ST, Gatley SJ. Imaging of the brain cannabinoid system. *Handb Exp Pharmacol.* 2005;168:425–443.

Linzen DH, Dingemans PM, Lenoir ME. Cannabis abuse and the course of recent onset schizophrenia disorders. *Arch General Psychiatry.* 1994;51:273–279.

Liu B-Q et al. Emerging tobacco hazards in China: 1. Retrospective proportional mortality study of one million deaths. *BMJ*. 1998;317:1411–1422.

Ludlow FH. *The Hasheesh Eater: Being Passages from the Life of a Pyathagorean.* New York: Harper Bros; 1857.

Lupica CR, Riegel AC, Hoffman AF. Marijuana and cannabinoid regulation of brain reward circuits. *Br J Pharmacol.* 2004;143:227–234.

Maccarrone M, Finazzi-Agrò A. Anandamide hydrolase: a guardian angel of human reproduction? *Trends Pharmacol Sci.* 2004;25:353–357.

Maccarrone M, Wenger T. Effects of cannabinoids on hypothalamic and reproductive function. *Handb Exp Pharmacol.* 2005;168:556–571.

MacCoun R, Reuter P. Interpreting Dutch cannabis policy: reasoning by analogy in the legalization debate. *Science.* 1997;278:47–52.

Mackie K. Distribution of cannabinoid receptors in the central and peripheral nervous system. *Handb Exp Pharmacol.* 2005;168:300–325.

Mackie K. Cannabinoid receptors as therapeutic targets. *Ann Rev Pharmacol Toxicol.* 2006;46:101–122.

Macleod J, Oakes R, Copello A, et al. Psychological and social sequelae of cannabis and other illicit drug use by young people: a systematic review of longitudinal, general population studies. *Lancet.* 2004;363:1579–1588.

Makriyannis A, Rapaka R. The molecular basis of cannabinoid activity. *Life Sci.* 1990;47:2173–2184.

Marshall CR. The active principle of Indian Hemp: a preliminary communication. *Lancet.* 1897;i:235–238.

Marsicano G, Wotjak CT, Azad SC, et al. The endogenous cannabinoid system controls extinction of aversive memories. *Nature.* 2002;418:488–489.

Martin BR. Characterization of the antinociceptive activity of $\Delta^9$-tetrahydrocannabinol in mice. In: Harvey DJ (ed). *Marihuana '84.* Oxford: IRL Press; 1985:685–692.

Matsuda LA, Lolait SJ, Brownstein MJ, Young AC, Bonner TI. Structure of a cannabinoid receptor and functional expression of the cloned cDNA. *Nature.* 1990;346:561–564.

Matthew RJ, Wilson WH, Coleman RE, Turkington TG, DeGrado TR. Marijuana intoxication and brain activation in marijuana smokers. *Life Sci.* 1997;60:2075–2089.

Matthew RJ, Wilson WH, Turkington TG, Coleman RE. Cerebellar activity and disturbed time sense after THC. *Brain Res.* 1998;797:183–189.

Matthias P, Tashkin DP, Marques-Magallanes JA, et al. Effects of varying marijuana potency on deposition of tar and delta-9-THC in the lung during smoking. *Pharmacol Biochem Behav.* 1997;58:1145–1150.

Mayor La Guardia's Committee on Marihuana. *The Marihuana Problem in the City of New York.* Lancaster, PA: J. Cattell Press; 1944.

Mechoulam R. Marihuana chemistry. *Science.* 1970;168:1159–1163.

Mechoulam R, Fride E, Di Marzo V. Endocannaninoids. *Eur J Pharmacol.* 1998;359:1–18.

Mechoulam R, Hanu L. A historical overview of chemical research on cannabinoids. *Chem Physics Lipids.* 2000;108:1–13.

Mehra R, Moore BA, Crothers K, Tetrault J, Fiellin DA. The association between marijuana smoking and lung cancer. *Arch Intern Med.* 2006;166:1359–1367.

Melges FT, Tinklenberg JR, Hollister LE, Gillespie HK. Marihuana and the temporal span of awareness. *Arch Gen Psychiatry.* 1971;24:564–567.

Moon JB. Sir William Brooke O'Shaugnessy—the foundations of fluid therapy and the Indian telegraph service. *New Engl J Med.* 1967;276:283–284.

Moore TH, Zammit S, Lingford-Hughes A et al. Cannabis use and risk of psychotic or affective mental health outcomes: a systematic review. *Lancet.* 2007; 370:319–328.

Morton GJ, Cummings DE, Baskin DG, et al. Central nervous system control of food intake and body weight. *Nature.* 2006;443:289–295.

Nadelmann EA. An end to marijuana prohibition. The drive to legalize picks up. *National Review.* 2004;July 12.

Nagayama T, Sinor AD, Simon RP, et al. Cannabinoids and neuroprotection in global and focal ischemia and in neuronal cultures. *J Neurosci.* 1999;19:2987–2995.

Nahas G. *Keep Off the Grass.* New York: Reader's Digest Press; 1976.

Nahas G. *Marihuana—Deceptive Weed.* New York: Raven Press; 1973.

Nahas G, Suciv-Foca G, Armand J-P, Morishima A. Inhibition of cellular mediated immunity in marihuana smokers. *Science.* 1974;183:419–420.

National Commission on Marihuana and Drug Abuse, First Report. *Marihuana: A Signal of Misunderstanding,* 1972, and Second Report, *Drug Use in America: Problem in Perspective,* 1973. Washington DC: US Government Printing Office. Available at: http://www.druglibrary.org/schaffer/Library/studies/nc/ncmenu.htm.

National Institutes of Health. *Report on the Medical Uses of Marijuana.* Bethesda, MD: National Institutes of Health; 1997.

Navarro M, et al. Acute administration of the $CB_1$ cannabinoid receptor antagonist SR141716A induces anxiety-like response in the rat. *NeuroReport.* 1997;8:491–496.

Negrete JC, Knapp WP, Douglas DE, Smith WB. Cannabis affects the severity of schizophrenic symptoms: results of a clinical survey. *Psychol Med.* 1986;16:515–520.

Nurmikko TJ, Serpell MJ, Hoggart B, Toomey PJ, Morlion BJ, Haines D. Sativex successfully treats neuropathic pain characterized by allodynia: a randomized, double-blind, placebo-controlled trial. *Pain,* 2007 (in press).

Okie S. Medical marijuana and the Supreme Court. *New Engl J Med.* 2005;353: 648–651.

Osei-Hyiaman D, DePetrillo M, Pacher P, et al. Endocannabinoid activation of hepatic CB-1 receptors stimulates fatty acid synthesis and contributes to diet-induced obesity. *J Clin Invest.* 2005;115:1298–1305.

O'Shaugnessey WB. On the preparation of the Indian hemp, or gunjah (cannabis indica) and their effects on the animal system in health and their utility in the treatment of tetanus and other convulsive disorders. *Trans Med Phys Soc Calcutta.* 1842;8:421–461.

Ossebaard HC. Netherlands' cannabis policy. *Lancet.* 1996;347:767–768.

Pacher P, Bátkai S, Kunos G. Cardiovascular pharmacology of cannabinoids. *Handb Exp Pharmacol.* 2005;168:600–625.

Paria BC, Dey SK. Ligand-receptor signalling with endocannabinoids in preimplantation embryo development and implantation. *Chem Phys Lipids.* 2000;108:211–220.

Pate DW, Jarvinen K, Urtti A, Mahadevan V, Jarvinen T. Effect of the CB1 receptor antagonist, SR141716A on cannabinoid-induced ocular hypotension in normotensive rabbits. *Life Sci.* 1998;63:2181–2188.

Pério A, Rimaldi-Carmona M, Maruani J, Barth F, Le fur G, Soubrié P. Central mediation of the cannabinoid cue: activity of a selective CB1 antagonist, SR 141716A. *Behav Pharmacol.* 1996;7:65–71.

Pert CB, Snyder SH. Opiate receptor demonstration in nervous tissue. *Science.* 1973;179:1011–1014.

Pertwee RG. Tolerance to and dependence on psychotropic cannabinoids. In: Pratt J (ed). *The Biological Basis of Drug Tolerance.* London: Academic Press Ltd; 1991:231–265.

Pertwee RG. The pharmacology and therapeutic potential of cannabidiol. In: Di Marzo V (ed). *Cannabinoids.* New York: Kluwer Academic/Plenum Publishers; 2004:32–83.

Pertwee RG (ed). Cannabinoids. *Handb Exp Pharmacol.* 2005a;168:1–770.

Pertwee RG. Pharmacological actions of cannabinoids. *Handb Exp Pharmacol.* 2005b;168:1–52.

Pettit DA, Harrison MP, Olsen JM, Spencer RF, Cabral GA. Immunohistochemical localization of the neural cannabinoid receptor in rat brain. *J Neurosci Res.* 1998;51:391–402.

Peto R. Influence of dose and duration of smoking on lung cancer rates. In: Zaridze DG, Peto R (eds). *Tobacco: A Major International Health Hazard.* Publication No 74. Lyon, France: International Agency for Research on Cancer; 1986:23–33.

Peto R, Lopez AD, Boreham J, Thun M, Heath Jr C, Doll R. Mortality from smoking worldwide. *Br Med Bull.* 1996;52:12–21.

Pijlman FT, Rigter SM, Hoek J, et al. Strong increase in total delta-THC in cannabis preparations sold in Dutch coffee shops. *Addict Biol.* 2005;10:171–180.

Piomelli D. The molecular logic of endocannabinoid signalling. *Nat Rev Neurosci.* 2003;4:873–884.

Piomelli D. The endocannabinoid system: a drug discovery perspective. *Curr Opin Invest Drugs.* 2005;6:672–679.

Piomelli V, Tarzia G, Duranti A, et al. Pharmacological profile of the selective FAAH inhibitor KDS-4103 (URB597). *CNS Drug Rev.* 2006;12:21–38.

Pi-Sunyer FX, Aronne LJ, Heshmati HM, et al. Effect of rimonabant, a cannabinoid-1 receptor blocker, on weight and cardiometabolic risk factors in overweight obese patients. *JAMA.* 2006;295:761–775.

Plasse TF, Gorter RW, Krasnow SH, Lane M, Shepard KV, Wadleigh RG. Recent clinical experience with dronabinol. *Pharmacol Biochem Behav.* 1991;40:695–700.

Polen MR, Sidney S, Tekawa IS, Sadler M, Friedman GD. Health care use by frequent marijuana smokers who do not smoke tobacco. *West J Med.* 1993;158:596–601.

Police Foundation. *Drugs and the Law.* London: Police Foundation; 2000.

Pope HG, Gruber AJ, Hudson JI, et al. Neuropsychological performance in long-term cannabis users. *Arch Gen Psychiatry.* 2001a;58:909–915.

Pope HG, Ionescu-Pioggia M, Pope KW. Drug use and life style among college undergraduates: a 30-year longitudinal study. *Am J Psychiatry.* 2001b;158:1519–21.

Porter AC, Sauer JM, Knierman MD, et al. Characterization of a novel endocannabinoid, virodhamine, with antagonist activity at the CB-1 receptor. *J Pharmacol Exp Ther.* 2002;301:1020–1024.

Pryce G, Baker D. Emerging properties of cannabinoid medicines in management of multiple sclerosis. *Trends Neurosci.* 2005;28:272–276.

Randall MC, Kendall DA, O'Sullivan S. The complexities of the cardiovascular actions of cannabinoids. *Br J Pharmacol.* 2004;142:20–26.

Reinarman C, Cohen PDA, Kaal HL. the limited relevance of drug policy: cannabis in Amsterdam and in San Francisco. *Am J Public Health.* 2004;94:836–842.

Reynolds JR. On the therapeutic uses and toxic effects of cannabis indica. *Lancet.* 1890;i:637–638.

Riedel G, Davies SN. Cannabinoid function in learning, memory and plasticity. *Handb Exp Pharmacol.* 2005;168:445–477.

Rinaldi-Carmona M, Barth F, Héauim M, et al. SR141716A, a potent and selective antagonist of the cannabinoid receptor. *FEBS Lett.* 1994;350:240–244.

Robbe H. Marijuana's impairing effects on driving are moderate when taken alone but severe when combined with alcohol. *Human Psychopharmacol.* 1998;13:S70–S78.

Robinson R. *The Great Book of Hemp.* Rochester, VT: Park Street Press; 1996.

Robson P. Human studies of cannabinoids and medicinal cannabis. *Handb Exp Pharmacol.* 2005;168:719–756.

Roffman R, Stephens S, eds. *Cannabis Dependence. Its Nature, Consequences and Treatment.* International Research Monographs in Addictions. Cambridge: Cambridge University Press; 2006.

Rog DJ, Nurmikko TJ, Friede T, Young CA. Randomized, controlled trial of cannabis-based medicine in central pain in multiple sclerosis. *Neurology.* 2005;65:812–819.

Royal College of Physicians. Cannabis and Cannabis-based Medicines. Available at: http://www.rcplondon.ac.uk; 2005.

Rubin V (ed). Cannabis and Culture. The Hague: Mouton Publishers; 1975.

Russo E. Cannabis for migraine treatment: the once and future prescription? An historical and scientific review. *Pain.* 1998;76:3–8.

Russo E. History of cannabis and its preparations in saga, science and sobriquet. *Chem Biodiversity.* 2007;4:1614–1648.

Sánchez C, Galve-Roperh I, Canova C, et al. Delta-9-tetrahydrocannabinol induces apoptosis in C6 glioma cells. *FEBS Lett.* 1998;436:6–10.

Sañudo-Peña MC, Tsou K, Walker JM. Motor actions of cannabinoids in the basal ganglia output nuclei. *Life Sci.* 1999;65:703–713.

Satz P, Fletcher JM, Sutker LS. Neurophysiologic, intellectual and personality correlates of chronic marijuana use in native Costa Ricans. *Ann NY Acad Sci.* 1976;282:266–306.

Scallet AC. Neurotoxicology of cannabis and THC: a review of chronic exposure studies in animals. *Pharmacol Biochem Behav.* 1991;40:671–676.

Semple DM, McIntosh AM, Lawrie SM. Cannabis as risk factor for psychosis: systematic review. *J Psychopharmacol.* 2005;19:187–194.

Serpell MG, Nurmikko T, Wright S. Long-term treatment of peripheral neuropathic pain with a phytocannabinoid medicine (Sativex). [Abstract] British Pain Society Meeting, Glasgow, March 30–April 1, 2006.

Serpell MG, Nurmikko TJ, Hoggart B, Toomey PJ, Morlion BJ. A multi-centre double blind, randomised, placebo-controlled trial of oromucosal cannabis based medicine in the treatment of neuropathic pain characterised by allodynia [Abstract]. UK Pain Society Meeting, Edinburgh, March 8–11, 2005.

Shen M, Thayer SA. Cannabinoid receptor agonists protect cultured rat hippocampal neurons from excitotoxicity. *Mol Pharmacol.* 1998;54:459–462.

Sidney S, Beck JE, Tekawa IS, Quesenberry CP, Friedman GD. Marijuana use and mortality. *Am J Public Health.* 1997;87:585–590.

Smiley A. Marijuana: on road and driving simulator studies. *Alcohol Drugs Driving.* 1986;2:121–134.

Smith AM, Fried PA, Hogan MJ, Cameron I. Effects of prenatal marijuana on visuospatial working memory: an fMRI study in young adults. *Neurotoxicol Teratol.* 2006;28:286–295.

Smith FL, Cichewicz D, Martin ZL, Welch SP. The enhancement of morphine antinociception in mice by delta-9-tetrahydrocannabinol. *Pharmacol Biochem Behav.* 1998;60:559–566.

Smith T, Smith H. Process for preparing cannabine or hemp resin. *Pharm J*. 1846;6:171-173.

Snyder SH. *Uses of Marijuana*. New York: Oxford University Press; 1971.

Solowij N. *Cannabis and Cognitive Functioning*. Cambridge: Cambridge University Press; 1998.

Steffens S, Vellard NR, Arnaud C, et al. Low dose oral cannabinoid therapy reduces progression of atherosclerosis in mice. *Nature*. 2005;434:782-786.

Swift W, Hall W, Teesson M. Cannabis use and dependence among Australian adults: results from the National Survey of Mental Health and Wellbeing. *Addiction*. 2001;96:737-748.

Szabo B, Schlicker E. Effects of cannabinoids on neurotransmission. *Handb Exp Pharmacol*. 2005;168:328-365.

Tanda G, Pontieri FE, Di Chiara G. Cannabinoid and heroin activation of mesolimbic dopamine transmission by a common $\mu_1$ opioid receptor mechanism. *Science*. 1997;276:2048-2050.

Tashkin DP. Smoked marijuana as a cause of lung injury. *Monalid Arch Chest Dis*. 2005;63:93-100.

Terranova JP, et al. Improvement of memory in rodents by the selective CB1 cannabinoid receptor antaognist, SR141716. *Psychopharmacology*. 1996;126:165-172.

Thakur GA, Nikas SP, Li C, Makryannis A. Structural requirements for cannabinoid receptor probes. *Handb Exp Pharmacol*. 2005;168:209-246.

Thirthalli J, Benegal V. Psychosis among substance users. *Curr Opin Psychiatry*. 2006;19:239-245.

Thomas H. Psychiatric symptoms in cannabis users. *Br J Psychiatry*. 1993;163:141-149.

Thornicroft G. Cannabis and psychosis. Is there epidemiological evidence for an association? *Br J Psychiatry*. 1990;157:25-33.

Todd AR. Hashish. *Experientia*. 1946;2:55-60.

Torbjörn U, Järbe C, Henriksson BG. Discriminative response control produced with hashish, tetrahydrocannabinols, and other drugs. *Psychopharmacology*. 1974;40:1-16.

Tramer MR, Carroll D, Campbell FA, et al. Cannabinoids for control of chemotherapy induced nausea and vomiting: quantitative systematic review. *BMJ*. 2001;323:16-21.

Valverde O, Karsak M, Zimmer A. Analysis of the endocannabinoid system by using $CB_1$ cannabinoid receptor knockout mice. *Handb Exp Pharmacol*. 2005;168:117-146.

Van Amsterdam JGC, van der Laan JW, Slangen JL. Residual effects of prolonged heavy cannabis use. Report No. 318902003. Bilthoven, Netherlands: National Institute of Public Health and the Environment; 1996.

Van Sickle MD, Duncan M, Kingsley PJ, et al. Identification and functional characterization of brainstem cannabinoid $CB_2$ receptors. *Science.* 2005;310:329–332.

Varma N, Carlson GC, Ledent C, Alger BE. Metabotropic glutamate receptors drive the endocannabinoid system in hippocampus. *J Neurosci.* 2001;21:RC188.

Vaughan VW, Christie MJ. Retrograde signalling by endocannabinoids. *Handb Exp Pharmacol.* 2005;168:368–383.

Wade D, Collin C, Stephens M. Meta-analysis of the effects of sativex on spasticity in MS subjects. *JMS Clin Lab Res.* 2005;11(Supp 1):S97.

Wade DT, Makela PM, House H, Bateman C, Robson P. Long-term use of a cannabis-based medicine in the treatment of spasticity and other symptoms in multiple sclerosis. *Mult Scler.* 2006;12:639–645.

Walker JM, Hohmann AG. Cannabinoid mechanisms of pain suppression. *Handb Exp Pharmacol.* 2005;168:511–544.

Walton RP. *Marihuana. America's New Drug Problem.* New York: J.B. Lippincott Co; 1938.

Wang H, Dey SK, Maccarrone M. Jekyll and Hyde: two faces of cannabinoid signalling in male and female fertility. *Endocrin Rev.* 2006;27:427–448.

Warburton H, May T, Hough M. Looking the other way. The impact of reclassifying cannabis on police warnings, arrests and informal action in England and Wales. *Br J Criminol.* 2005;45:113–128.

Ware MA, Adams H, Guy GW. The medicinal use of cannabis in the UK: results of a nationwide survey. *Int J Clin Pract.* 2005;59:291–295.

Weil AT, Zinberg NE, Nelsen JM. Clinical and psychological effects of marihuana in man. *Science.* 1968;162:1234–1242.

WHO. Cannabis: a Health Perspective and Research Agenda. 1997. Geneva, World Health Organization.

Wiley JL, Barret RL, Lowe J, Balster RL, Martin BR. Discriminative stimulus effects of CP55,940 and structurally dissimilar cannabinoids in rats. *Neuropharmacology.* 1995;34:669–676.

Williams JH, Wellman NA, Rawlins JNP. Cannabis use correlates with schizotypy in healthy people. *Addiction.* 1996;91:869–887.

Williams SJ, Hartley JPR, Graham JDP. Bronchodilator effects of delta-9-THC administered by aerosol to asthmatic patients. *Thorax.* 1976;31:720–723.

Wilson RI, Nicoll RA. Endogenous cannabinoids mediate retrograde signalling at hippocampal synapses. *Nature.* 2001;410:588–592.

Wisset R. *A Treatise on Hemp.* London: J. Harding; 1808.

Witkin JM, Tzavara ET, Davis RJ, Li X, Nomikos GG. A therapeutic role for cannabinoid CB-1 receptor antagonists in major depressive disorders. *Trends Pharmacol Sci.* 2005;26:609–617.

Wood GB, Bache F. *The Dispensatory of the United States.* Philadelphia: Lippincott; 1854:339.

Wu TC, Tashkin DP, Djaheb B, Rose JE. Pulmonary hazards of smoking marijuana as compared with tobacco. *New Engl J Med.* 1988;31:347–351.

Zajicek J, Fox P, Sanders H, et al. Cannabinoids for treatment of spasticity and other symptoms related to multiple sclerosis (CAMS study): multicentre randomised placebo-controlled trial. *Lancet.* 2003;362:1517–1526.

Zajicek JP, Sanders HP, Wright DE, et al. Cannabinoids in multiple sclerosis (CAMS study): safety and efficacy data for 12 months follow-up. *J Neurol Neurosurg Psychiatry.* 2005;76:1664–1669.

Zammit S, Allebeck P, Andreasson S, Lundberg I, Lewis G. Self reported cannabis use as a risk factor for schizophrenia in Swedish conscripts of 1969: historical cohort study. *BMJ.* 2002;325:1195–1212.

Zimmer A, Zimmer AM, Hohmann AG, Herkenham M, Bonner TI. Increased mortality, hypoactivity, and hypoalgesia in cannabinoid CB1 receptor knockout mice. *Proc Natl Acad Sci USA.* 1999;96:5780–5785.

Zimmer L, Morgan JP. *Marijuana Myths, Marijuana Facts.* New York: Lindesmith Center; 1997.

Ziring D, Wei B, Velazquez P, Schrage M, Buckley NE, Braun J. Formation of B and T cell subsets require the cannabinoid receptor CB2. *Immunogenetics.* 2006;58:714–725.

Zuardi AW, Crippa JAS, Hallak JEC, Moreira FA, Guimarães FS. Cannabidiol, a Cannabis sativa constituent, as an antipsychotic drug. *Braz J Med Biol Res.* 2006;39:421–429.

Zuardi AW, Shirakawa I, Finkelfarb E, Karniol IG. Action of cannabidiol on the anxiety and other effects produced by delta-9-THC in normal subjects. *Psychopharmacology.* 1982;76:245–250.

Zuckerman B, Frank DA, Hingson R, et al. Effects of maternal marijuana and cocaine use on fetal growth. *New Engl J Med.* 1989;320:762–768.

# Index

acetaminophen, endocannabinoid
    activation, 75
acetylcholine, delta-9-tetrahydrocannabinol
    inhibition, 57
Adams, Roger, 32–33
addiction
    recreational cannabis use and, 209–212
    tolerance and dependence and
        definitions of, 106–113
adenylate cyclase, cannabinoid inhibition
    of, 49
Advisory Council on the Misuse of Drugs,
    203–206
Africa, cannabis consumption in, 217
agonists, cannabinoid receptors, 52–54
AIDS infection, cannabis effects on, 171
AIDS wasting syndrome, cannabis for
    counteraction of, 129–130, 144–145
alcohol
    cannabis consumption with, 198–201,
        207–209
    cannabis effects compared with, 98–99
    cannabis preparations using, 16–17
    effects on driving of, 95–96
alkaloids, plant sources of, 28
AM404 anadamide analog, 75, 77–78
AM1172 analog, endocannabinoid
    inactivation inhibition, 78–79
*American Magazine*, 21
amide hydrolase family, endocannabinoid
    inactivation inhibition, 79

amotivational syndrome, cognitive deficits
    from long-term cannabis use and,
    166–167
anandamide
    AM404 anadamide inhibition, 78–79
    development of, 69
    endocannabinoid biosynthesis and
        inactivation, 70–72
    pain sensitivity, 75
animal studies
    antiepileptic effects of cannabis, 145–146
    cannabis effects, 99–104
    cannabis toxicity, 159–162
    medicinal uses of cannabis
        multiple sclerosis and, 133–137
        pain management, 138–141
    of tolerance and dependence on
        cannabis, 105–113
Anslinger, Harry J., 21, 25, 223, 225–227
antagonists for cannabinoids, development
    of, 39–41
antiepileptic medicines, cannabis as,
    145–146
aphrodisiac claims for cannabis, 116–117
appetite stimulation, uses of cannabis for,
    144–115
aprepitant (Emend), anti-emetic effects of,
    144
Arab civilizations
    history of cannabis in, 19–22
    medicinal use of cannabis in, 116–117

2-Arachidonylglycerol (2-AG)
  endocannabinoid biosynthesis, 71–72
  isolation of, 69–70
  arachidonic acid, endocannabinoid
    biosynthesis and inactivation, 70–72
Arnold of Lübeck, 21
art, cannabis intoxication and perceptions
  of, 88–89
Ashton, Heather, 201–202
Ashworth scale, cannabis therapy for
  multiple sclerosis and, 134–137
Assassins mythology, 20–21
Assyrian civilization, hemp cultivation in,
  18–19
asthma, cannabis effects on, 146–147
atropine, plant sources of, 28
Australia
  decriminalization of cannabis in,
    239–241
  research on cannabis in, 230–231
autoimmune disorders, cannabis use for, 148

baclofen, multiple sclerosis therapy, 132
Baudelaire, Charles, 23–24, 83
benzodiazepines, cannabis dependency and
  tolerance compared with, 109–113
Berke, J., 84
β-interferon, multiple sclerosis therapy,
  131–132
bhang (herbal cannabis)
  ancient Indian references to, 18
  Arabian references to, 19
  Indian consumption of, 215–216,
    224–225
  medicinal uses of, 116–117
  preparation of, 16–17
Billy Martin tetrad
  cannabinoid effects correlation, 64–65
  endocannabinoids, 69
binding assays, cannabinoid receptor activity
  and, 51–52
biochemical models, cannabis receptors, 52
biosynthesis, endocannabinoids, 70–72
bladder control, medicinal use of cannabis
  in, 132–137

Blue Velvet Coffee Shop (Amsterdam), 4
Blunkett, David, 236
blunts, cannabis consumption using,
  192–195
body weight, endocannabinoids and, 74
bongs, for marijuana smoking, 15–16
brain
  cannabinoid neurotransmission in, 48–50
  cannabis effects on
    dependency and tolerance and,
      110–113
    functional impairment, 96–99,
      161–162
    gateway effects, 209
    psychotropic effects, 84–94
  chemical messenger-system in, ix–x
  cognitive deficits from long-term
    cannabis use in, 164–167
  delta-9-tetrahydrocannabinol delivery to,
    41–47
  neuroanatomical distribution of CB-1
    receptors in, 54–56
Brazil, cannabis consumption in, 219
British Pharmacopoiea, 26
  cannabis in, 119–120
bronchitis, cannabis use and, 185–186

California, hemp cultivation in, 6
Callaghan, James, 228–229
Cambodia, cannabis consumption in,
  216–217
Canada
  cannabis cultivation in, 193–195
  medicinal use of cannabis in, 4
  research on cannabis in, 230–231
cancer
  cannabis for pain management with,
    140–141
  cannabis therapy for, 148
  chemotherapy-induced vomiting,
    cannabis for, 141–144
cannabidiol
  antiseizure activity of, 146
  binding assays of, 52
  chemical properties of, 32–33, 35

receptor mechanisms in, 53–54
cannabin, development of, 29
cannabinoid receptors
    agonists and antagonists, 77, 151–155
    antiseizure activity, 145–146
    discovery of, 48–54
    neuroanatomical distribution in brain,
        54–56
    tolerance and dependence and role of,
        105–113
cannabinoids
    agonists and antagonists, 39–41, 151–155
    animal studies of effects of, 100–104
    anti-inflammatory actions, 148
    defined, 68
    medicinal applications, 128–130
    natural sources of, 32–33
    neuroprotective effects of, 161–162
    synthetic forms of, 36–39
    toxicity studies of, 161–162
cannabinol, isolation and chemical
        structure, 29–33
cannabis. *See also* hemp plant *(Cannabis
        sativa)*
    acute effects of, 162–164
    age levels for recreational use of, 189–191
    alcohol effects compared with, 98–99
    animal studies of effects, 99–104
    autoimmune disorders therapy and, 148
    cancer therapy, 148
    central nervous system effects, 82–113
    cognitive deficits from long-term use,
        164–167
    diarrhea, 148
    eating and drinking of, 16–17
    fertility and pregnancy effects, 168–170
    forensic testing for, 212–214
    future research about, 222–242
    as gateway drug, 206–209, 233–238
    global statistics on recreational use,
        188–189
    history of, 17–26
    immune system suppression, 170–171
    laboratory studies with human volunteers,
        94–99

learning and memory effects of, 96–98
long-term exposure effects, 164–175
medicinal applications of, 4, 116–156,
    ix–xi
mental illness and, 171–175
movement and driving effects of, 95–96
oil, extraction of, 11
preparations of, 10, 14–18
prevalence of use, 189–192
recreational use of, 188–220
research issues concerning, i–ix
resin
    extraction and purification, 28–29
    extraction of, 10–11
    medicinal uses of, 116–117
    smoking of, 15–16
    sources of, 193–195
safety of, 158–186
statistics on use of, 4
storage of, 28
supply sources for, 192–195
tolerance and dependence, studies of,
    105–113, 167–168
toxicity of, 158–162
varieties of, 7
*Cannabis and Cognitive Functioning*, 167
*Cannabis Experience, The*, 84
cannabis-induced psychological stress
    syndrome (CIPDS), 241
Cannabis in Multiple Sclerosis (CAMS)
    therapy, 133–137
cannabis psychosis, 163–164
Cannabis Tax Act of 1937, 25–26,
    225–226
cardiovascular system
    cannabis effects on, 164, 185–186
    endocannabinoids and, 76
Caribbean
    cannabis consumption in, 217–218
    cannabis cultivation in, 192–195
    history of cannabis use in, 25
Carter, Jimmy, 230–231
casual recreational cannabis use, defined,
    196–198
catalepsy, cannabinoids and, 61–63

catechol-O-methyl transferase (COMT),
    cannabis use and, 173–175
CB-1 receptor
    agonists and antagonists, 77
    animal studies of, 102–104
    cannabis use for multiple sclerosis
        therapy, 132–137
    cardiovascular control and, 76
    development of, 39–41
    discovery of, 52–54
    endocannabinoids and, 69–70, 78–79
    energy metabolism and body weight
        and, 74
    heart and blood vessel effects and, 58–59
    medicinal uses of cannabis and, 130
    mood disorders and sleep therapy and,
        147
    motility and posture effects, 62–63
    neuroanatomical distribution in brain,
        54–56
    neurotransmitter inhibition, 56–57
    pain sensitivity and, 59–61
    reproductive system effects, 76–77
    retrograde signal molecules, 72–74
    tolerance and dependence on cannabis
        and role of, 109–113
CB-2 receptor
    agonists and antagonists, 77
    cardiovascular control and, 76
    development of, 39–41
    discovery of, 52–54
    endocannabinoids and, 69–70
    immune system function and, 170–171
    pain sensitivity and, 60–61
central nervous system (CNS)
    animal studies of cannabinoid effects in,
        100–104
    cannabinoid effects on, 60–61
    cannabis effects on, 82–113
    medicinal uses of cannabis and, 131–132
charas (cannabis resin), 15–16, 215–216
chillum, Indian consumption of, 215–216
China, hemp cultivation in, 17–18
cholera, early research on, 118
Chronica Slavorum, 21

cisplatin-induced nausea and vomiting,
    cannabis for management of,
        141–144
clinical trials
    cannabis-based multiple sclerosis therapy,
        132–137
    medicinal uses of cannabis, 4, 126–128
    rimonabant, 152–155
Club des Hashischins (Paris), 22–23
cocaine
    cannabis as gateway drug to, 206–209
    isolation and extraction from coca, 28
cognitive deficits
    long-term cannabis use and, 164–167
    prenatal effects of cannabis and, 169
Colombia
    cannabis consumption in, 219
    supply sources for, 192–195
consumption of cannabis
    in Africa, 217
    Caribbean and Latin America, 217–218
    eating and drinking of, 16–17
    global patterns of, 214–219
    incidence of, 198–201
    in India, 215–216
    in Nepal and Tibet, 216
    smoking of, 14–16
    sources and forms of, 192–195
    in Southeast Asia, 216–217
    statistics on, 189–192
CP55,940 synthetic cannabinoid
    animal studies of effects of, 100–104
    binding assays of, 51–54
    neuroprotective effects of, 161
Culpepper, Nicholas, 117
cultivation of cannabis, 192–195
    in Jamaica, 217–218
    potency increases and, 202–206
cyclic adenosine monophosphate (cAMP),
    cannabinoid inhibition of, 49–50

dagga (African cannabis), 217
decriminalization of cannabis
    case for, 238–241
    future research on, 222–242

in Netherlands, 232–238
*Deer Hunter, The,* 188
delta-9-tetrahydrocannabinol (THC)
    animal studies of effects of, 100–104
    artificial hemp cultivation and, 11–13
    asthma treament use, 146–147
    Billy Martin tetrad and effects of, 64–65
    brain delivery systems for, 41–47
    cancer therapy, 148
    eating and drinking of, 16–17
    elimination of, 47–48
    emerging research on, x–xi
    forensic testing of, 212–214
    gateway drug use and, 207–209
    generic name (dronabinol), 129–130
    heart and blood vessel effects of, 57–59
    hemp cultivation and increased yields
        of, 6–12
    herbal cannabis, 203–206
    human laboratory studies of, 94–99
    isolation of, 29–36
    in marijuana joints, 14–16
    medicinal use of, 129–130
    mood disorders and sleep therapy, 147
    motility and posture effects, 61–63
    multiple sclerosis therapy, 1320136
    neurotransmitter inhibition of, 56–57
    oral absorption of, 43–47
    pain sensitivity and effects of, 59–61
    persistence in body of, 47–48
    pharmacology, 28–65
    physiological effects of, 56–65
    plant sources of, 193–195
    potency levels of, 201–206
    psychoactive effects of, 48–49, 84–94
    receptors, discovery of, 50–54
    recreational use patterns and, 196–198
    smoking as delivery route for, 41–43
    synthetic analogs, 36–39
    tobacco smoke and, 176–185
    toxicity studies of, 159–162
    transmission mechanisms for, 49–50
    U.S. prison experiments on, 225–226
De Nerval, Gerard, 22
dependency

    DSM-IV substance dependence criteria
        for, 107–108
    long-term cannabis use and development
        of, 105–113, 167–168
    recreational cannabis use and,
        209–212
depolarization-induced suppression of
    inhibition (DSI), retrograde signal
    molecules, 73–74
depressant effects, of cannabinoids, 61–63
depression, cannabis for treatment of, 123
diacylglycerol (DAG), endocannabinoid
    biosynthesis and inactivation, 70–72
diarrhea, cannabis treatment for, 121, 148
diazepam, multiple sclerosis therapy, 132
dopamine
    cannabis dependency and tolerance and,
        110–113
    delta-9-tetrahydrocannabinol
        neurotransmitter stimulation of, 57
dose levels
    psychotropic effects of cannabis and,
        82–83
    tar deposition from smoked marijuana
        and, 178–185
double consciousness, cannabis
    intoxication and, 91
driving, cannabis effects on, 95–96
dronabinol (marinol)
    anti-emetic effects of, 142–144
    appetite stimulation with, 145
    medical uses of, 129–130
    oral administration of, 45–46
drug delivery mechanisms
    alternative routes for cannabis delivery,
        46–47
    delta-9-tetrahydrocannabinol, 41–47
    DSM-IV diagnostic criteria, dependency
        and tolerance, 107–108, 211–212
Dumas, Alexander, 22, 83
dysentery, cannabis treatment for, 121

Egypt, history of cannabis in, 21–22
elimination, of delta-9-tetrahydrocannabinol
    from body, 47–48

endocannabinoids
  biosynthesis and inactivation of, 70–72
  cardiovascular effects, 76
  energy metabolism and body weight
    control, 74
  inactivation inhibitors, 77–79
  natural sources of, 68–70
  pain sensitivity, 74–75
  pharmacology, 77–79
  physiological functions, 72–77
  receptor agonists and antagonists, 77
  reproductive effects, 76–77
  retrograde signal molecules at synapses,
    72–74
endorphins
  current research on, ix–x
  delta-9-tetrahydrocannabinol
    neurotransmitter stimulation of, 57
  endocannabinoids and, 68
  pain sensitivity and effects of
    cannabinoids, 59–61
energy metabolism, endocannabinoids
  and, 74
environmental factors, in cannabis
  intoxication, 83
epilepsy, cannabis as anticonvulsant,
  117–118, 145–146
Europe
  history of cannabis in, 22–23
  legalization of cannabis in, 5
  medicinal uses of cannabis in, 117
European Monitoring Centre for Drugs and
  Drug Addiction, 12
European Union (EU)
  cannibis transportation and, 5
  hemp farming policies from, 14
experimental cannabis users, prevalence of,
  190–192

fantasies, cannabis intoxication and
  experiences with, 90–91
fatty acid amide hydrolase (FAAH)
  endocannabinoid biosynthesis, 71–72
  endocannabinoid inactivation inhibition,
    77–78

retrograde signal molecules, 72–74
fatty acids, endocannabinoid biosynthesis
  and inactivation, 70–72
fatuous euphoria, effects of cannabis as, 86
fertility, cannabis impact on, 168–169
Fields, Howard, 124–125
fluid replacement therapy, cholera, 118
fluoxetine, endocannabinoid
  biosynthesis, 72
folk medicine, cannabis use and, 124–128
forensic cannabis testing, growth of,
  212–214
fractional distillation, cannabis resin
  extraction and, 29
France, history of cannabis in, 22–23

Galen, on cannibis consumption, 19
γ-aminobutyric acid (GABA)
  delta-9-tetrahydrocannabinol inhibition,
    57, 61–63
  medicinal uses of cannabis and, 132
ganja
  consumption patterns for, 215–218
  extraction of, 29
  hemp cultivation and extraction of, 10
  medicinal uses of, 116–117
  smoking of, 15–16
Garvey, Marcus, 217–218
gateway drug, cannabis as, 206–209, 233–238
Gautier, Pierre, 22–23, 83
genetics, cannabis receptor research and,
  52–54
Goode, E., 84, 87
GPR55 cannabinoid receptor, development
  of, 54
Great Britain
  cannabis dependency in, 211–212
  cannabis therapy for multiple sclerosis
    in, 134–137
  decriminalization of cannabis in,
    235–241
  gateway drug use and, 207–209
  history of hemp cultivation in, 23–24
  Indian cannabis investigations by,
    223–225

legalization of cannabis in, 5
medicinal use of cannabis in, 26,
  118–120
recreational cannabis use in, 195–198
research on cannabis in, 227–229
Greek civilization, hemp cultivation and
  use in, 19

Haile Selassie, 217–218
hallucinations, cannabis intoxication and,
  89–90
Hasan, Khwaja A., 15
Hasan-Ibn-Sabbah, 20–21
*Hasheesh Eater, The*, 24, 83–84
hashish
  Arabian historical references to, 19–22
  from cannibis resin, 10–11
  delta-9-tetrahydrocannabinol extraction
    from, 33–35
  medicinal uses of, 116–117
  psychotropic effects of, 84–94
Hayder (Sufi founder), 19
*Health and Psychological Consequences of
  Cannabis Use, The*, 222
heart, cannabinoid effects on, 57–59
heavy recreational cannabis use, defined,
  197–198
hemp plant *(Cannabis sativa)*
  agricultural products from, 13–14
  artificial cultivation of, 11–13
  botanical characteristics, 6
  cataleptic effects of, 61–63
  cultivation of, 7–12
  food crops from, 13
  history of cultivation of, 17–24
  medicinal uses of, 117
  seed suppliers for, 7
herbal medicine, cannabis use and, 124–128
Hernton, C. H., 84
heroin
  cannabis as gateway drug to, 206–209
  cannabis dependency and tolerance
    compared with, 110–113
Himmelstein, Jerome, 227
hippocampus

animal studies of cannabis effects on, 104
  cannabis toxicity and, 161–162
homeopathic medicine
  cannabis use and, 124–128
  medicinal use of cannabis in, 120–122
horror, as cannabis side-effect, 92–94
Hugo, Victor, 22–23
hydroponic cannabis, potency of, 204–206
11-hydroxy-tetrahydrocannabinol
    metabolite
  formation of, 44–45
  medicinal uses of cannabis and, 129–130
hypothalamus, cannabis effects on, 169

illicit marijuana, potency of, 201–206
immune system function, cannabis effects
  on, 170–171
immunohistochemical mapping
  endocannabinoid biosynthesis, 71–72
  neuroanatomical distribution of CB-1
    receptors, 54–56
Independent Drug Monitoring Unit
    (IDMU)
  cannabis cultivation, 193–195
  recreational cannabis use and,
    195–201
India
  cannabis consumption patterns in,
    15–16, 215–216
  cannabis-containing food and drink in,
    16–17
  hemp cultivation and cannabis extraction
    in, 10–11
  history of cannabis use in, 18–19
  investigations of cannabis in, 223–225
  medicinal use of cannabis in, 116–122
  safety studies on cannabis in, 171–172
Indian Hemp Drugs Commission Report,
    18, 171–172, 215–216, 223–225
inhalation aerosols
  cannabis use in, 146–147
  delta-9-tetrahydrocannabinol delivery
    through, 46–47
inhalation volumes, delta-9-tetrahydro-
    cannabinol delivery to brain, 41–43

Institute of Medicine, 123–124
Internet, cannabis information sources on,
    193–195
intoxication
    characteristics of, in cannabis, 84–94,
        163–164
    dose levels of cannabis and intensity of,
        82–83
intravenous drug delivery
    cannabis insolubility as barrier to, 42–43
    medicinal uses of cannabis and, 121–122
inverse agonists
    cannabinoid receptors, 52–54
    pain sensitivity and, 60–61

Jamaica, cannabis consumption in, 217–218
Japan, medicinal uses of cannabis in,
    121–122
*Journal of the American Medical Association*
    (JAMA), 227

*Keep Off the Grass*, 231
kif (African cannabis), 217
*kunnubu/kunnapu* (ancient reference to
    hemp), 18–19

laboratory studies of cannabis effects,
    human volunteers, 94–99
La Dain Report, 230–231
La Guardia, Fiorello, 225–231
*Lancet, The*, 239
Laos, cannabis consumption in, 216–217
Latin America
    cannabis consumption in, 217–218
    history of cannabis use in, 25
League of Nations Convention on Narcotic
    Control (1925), 222
learning function, cannabis effects on,
    96–98
legalization of cannabis
    propositions for, 4
    U.S. opposition to, 5
*Les Paradis Artificiels*, 23–24
Levine, Jon, 124–125
levonantradol, development of, 37–39

L-glutamate, endocannabinoid biosynthesis,
    70–72
Livet, Louis, 219
long-term cannabis exposure, cognitive
    deficits from, 164–167
long-term depression (LTD), depolarization-
    induced suppression of inhibition and,
    73–74
long-term potentiation, animal studies of
    cannabis effects on, 104
Ludlow, Fitz Hugh, 24, 83–85, 88–94
lung cancer, cannabis inhalation and,
    181–185
lungs, smoked marijuana effects on,
    179–185

macrophage studies, of smoked marijuana,
    180–185
Marco Polo, 20
*Marihuana—Deceptive Weed*, 231
marijuana. *See* cannabis
marijuana high, subjective reports on,
    82–94
marijuana joint
    characteristics of, 14–16
    sources and preparation of, 192–195
*Marijuana Myths, Marijuana Facts*, 158
marijuana psychosis, 163–164
*Marijuana Smokers, The*, 84e
Marijuana Tax Act (U.S.), 25–26, 223
marinol
    development of, 45–46
    medicinal uses of, 129–130
Marley, Bob, 218
Marshall, C. R. (Dr.), 29–31
McCaffrey, Barry, 123
Mechoulam, Raphael, 34, 68–69
medicinal uses of cannabis
    AIDS wasting syndrome, 144–145
    bronchial asthma, 146–147
    cancer, 148
    clinical trials on, 4
    diarrhea, 148
    disease and medical conditions targeted
        by, 131–148

emerging possible applications, 148
epilepsy, 145–146
future research issues, 155–156
history of, 25–26, 116–122
modern interest in, 122–127
mood disorders and sleep, 147
multiple sclerosis, 131–137
obesity treatment, cannabinoid
    antagonists, 151–155
pain management, 137–144
smoked marijuana, 149–151
synthetic cannabinoids, 128–130
    dronabinol (marinol), 129–130
    nabilone (cesamet), 130
Melges, Frederick, 87–88
memory
    animal studies of cannabis effects on,
        102–104
    cannabis effects on, 96–98
    cognitive deficits from long-term
        cannabis use, 164–167
mental illness
    cannabis effects on, 163–164,
        171–175, 186
    cannabis use in treatment of, 120–122
metabolites
    elimination of delta-9-
        tetrahydrocannabinol and, 47–48
    forensic testing of cannabis and, 212–214
    oral absorption of delta-9-
        tetrahydrocannabinol and, 44–47
methanandamide, endocannabinoid
    biosynthesis, 71–72
Mexico, cannabis consumption in, 219
migraine, cannabis for pain management
    in, 141
military, recreational use of cannabis in,
    188
Misuse of Drugs Act of 1971, 26, 229, 235
Montgomery, Neil, 196–198
mood disorders, cannabis effects on, 147
mood states, cannabis effects on, 83
morbidity and mortality statistics, on
    cannabis use, 158–159
Moreau, Jean Jacques, 119–120

morphine, plant sources of, 28
motility, cannabinoid effects on, 61–63
motor function
    alcohol effects on, 98–99
    cannabis effects on, 95–96
multiple sclerosis (MS)
    AIDS wasting syndrome, 131–137
    cannabis for treatment of, 123
muscarine, mushroom sources of, 28
music, cannabis intoxication and
    perceptions of, 88–89

nabilone
    anti-emetic effects of, 142–144
    development of, 37–39
nabilone (cesamet), medicinal use of, 130
Nahas, Gabrial, 231
nantradol, development of, 37–39
Napoleon, history of cannabis and invasions
    by, 22
N-arachidonoyldopamine (NADA)
    isolation of, 70
    pain sensitivity, 75
natalizumab, multiple sclerosis therapy,
    131–132
National Commission on Marihuana and
    Drug Abuse (U.S.), 229–231
National Institute on Drug Abuse, 231
Native Americans, history of cannabis use
    among, 25
nausea
    cannabis for counteraction of, 129–130,
        141–144
    as cannabis side-effect, 91–92
Nepal, cannabis consumption in, 216
nerve injury, cannabis for pain management
    from, 140–141
Netherlands
    decriminalization of cannabis in, 232–241
    gateway drug use and, 207–209, 233–238
    hemp cultivation, 6
    legalization of cannabis in, 4–5
    medicinal use of cannabis in, 123
    potency levels of cannabis in, 202–206
    skunk production in, 195

neurodegenerative diseases, cannabis
    treatment for, 148
neuropathic pain syndromes, medicinal
    uses of cannabis and, 138–141
neuropathy, cannabis for treatment of, 123
neurotransmitters
    cannabinoid effects and, 49–50
    delta-9-tetrahydrocannabinol inhibition
        of, 56–57
New England Journal of Medicine, 168–169
New Homeopathic Pharmacopoeia
    and Posology or the Preparation of
    Homeopathic Medicine, 120
New Zealand, research on cannabis in,
    230–231
nicotine, cannabis mixed with, 176–185
Nixon, Richard M., 229–239
noradrenaline, delta-9-tetrahydrocannabinol
    inhibition, 57

obesity, cannabinoid antagonists and,
    151–155
Office of National Drug Control Policy
    (ONDCP), 238
Old Man of the Mountains, 20
Olsen, Carl, 218–219
opiate receptors, binding mechanisms of, 51
oral absorption mechanisms
    cannabis-based asthma therapy, 146–147
    delta-9-tetrahydrocannabinol, 43–47
    medicinal uses of cannabis, 129–130
    pain management, 138–141
organ bath assays, delta-9-
        tetrahydrocannabinol neurotransmitter
        inhibition, 57
O'Shaugnessy, William B., 11, 117–119

pain sensitivity
    cannabinoid effects on, 59–61
    endocannabinoids and, 74–75
    medicinal uses of cannabis, 137–141
    multiple sclerosis, 132–137
    self-medication with cannabis, 122–128
partial agonists, cannabinoid receptors,
    52–54

Pent-Ts'ao Kang Mu (Chinese herbal)
    hemp plant described in, 17–18
    medical uses of cannabis in, 116–122
personality traits, cannabis effects and, 83
Pertwee, Roger, 68–69
pharmaceutical industry, medicinal uses
    of cannabis and, 122, 130, 134–137,
    143–146
pipes, for marijuana smoking, 15–16
placebo effects
    medicinal uses of cannabis and, 124–128
    multiple sclerosis therapy, 136–137
plants, drug isolation and extraction from,
    28
Platoon, 188
pleasure and reward pathways,
    endocannabinoids and, 76–77
polm
    from hemp plants, 10
    production of, 193–195
popular culture, recreational use of
    cannabis in, 188
postural hypotension, as cannabinoid effect,
    58–59
posture, cannabinoid effects on, 61–63
potency levels
    illicit marijuana, 201–206
    psychotropic effects of cannabis and,
        82–83
    tar deposition from smoked marijuana
        and, 178–185
Potency Monitoring Project, 202–206
pravadoline, development of, 38–39
pregnancy, cannabis effects on, 168–169,
    185–186
prenatal effects of cannabis, 168–169
prevalence of cannabis use, statistics on,
    189–192
psychiatry, cannabis use in, 120–122
psychic distress, as cannabis side-effect,
    91–92
psychoactive drugs, consumer ratings of,
    200–201
psychomotor function
    cannabinoid effects on, 63, 163–164

long-term cannabis use and, 164–167
psychotropic effects of cannabis
  cannabis psychosis, 163–164
  mental illness and, 171–175
  subjective reports of, 82–94
public opinion, on decriminalization of
  cannabis, 238–241
puff volumes, delta-9-tetrahydrocannabinol
  delivery to brain, 41–43

quinine, plant sources of, 28

radioactive detection
  cannabinoid neurotransmission, 50–51
  neuroanatomical distribution of CB-1
    receptors, 54–56
Rastafarian movement, cannabis
  consumption in, 217–218
recreational cannabis use, 188–220
  dependency and, 209–212
  effects of, 198–201
  as gateway drug, 206–209
  patterns of, 195–198
  potency of illicit marijuana, 201–206
  prevalence statistics, 189–192
  production and consumption patterns,
    192–195
rectal suppositories, delta-9-
  tetrahydrocannabinol delivery through,
  46–47
reflex hypersensitivity, cannabinoids and,
  61–63
regular recreational cannabis use, defined,
  196–198
reproductive system
  cannabis impact on, 168–169
  endocannabinoids and, 76–77
retrograde signal molecules,
  endocannabinoids and, 72–74
Reynolds, John Russell, 119–120
rheumatoid arthritis, cannabis for treatment
  of, 123, 140–141
rimonabant
  agonist/antagonist activity, 77
  animal studies of, 102–104

depolarization-induced suppression of
  inhibition and, 73–74
development of, 39–41
effects on pain sensitivity of, 59–61
obesity management and, 151–155
tolerance and dependence on, 109–113
roach, characteristics of, 14–16
Runciman, Ruth, 235–236

safety issues with cannabis, 156–187
  acute effects, 162–164
  immune system function, 170–171
  impact on fertility and unborn children,
    168–170
  long-term use effects, 164–175
  lung cancer and, 181–185
  mental illness and, 171–175
  smoked marijuana hazards, 175–185
  tolerance and dependence potential,
    167–168
  toxicity effects, 158–162
Sativex plant extract
  cannabis delivery through, 46–47
  multiple sclerosis therapy, 135–137
  pain management, 139–141
schizophrenia, cannabis effects on,
  163–164, 171–175, 185–186
schizotypy, mental illness classification
  and, 173
school children, cannabis consumption by,
  226–231
Science of Charms, 18
second messenger systems, cannabinoid
  neurotransmission and, 49–50
self-medication, by marijuana users,
  122–128
sensimilla
  hemp cultivation and extraction of, 10
  smoking of, 15–16
serotonin, endocannabinoid biosynthesis, 72
sexual function
  cannabis impact on, 168–169
  recreational cannabis use and, 199–201
short-term memory, cannabis effects on,
  97–98

side-effects of cannabis
  dose levels and, 82–83
  recreational consumption patterns and,
    198–201
skunk, production of, 193–195
sleep
  aftermath of cannabis intoxication and,
    91–92
  cannabis effects on, 147
Smith, T. and H., 29
smoking
  cannabis ingestion through, 14–16
  delta-9-tetrahydrocannabinol delivery
    and, 41–43
  lung cancer and marijuana smoke,
    181–185
  lung effects of marijuana, 179–185
  medicinal use of cannabis and, 122,
    149–151
  special hazards of smoked marijuana,
    175–185
soap bar (cannabis resin), 193–195
Solowij, Nadia, 167
Southeast Asia, cannabis consumption in,
    216–217
spliffs, cannabis consumption through,
    193–195
Squire, Peter, 118
Strange Career of Marijuana, The, 227
stress, endocannabinoid activation, 75
strychnine, plant sources of, 28
substance dependence, DSM-IV criteria
    for, 107
synapses, retrograde signal molecules,
    72–74
synthetic cannabinoids, medicinal
    applications, 128–130
  dronabinol (marinol), 129–130
  nabilone (cesamet), 130

Tashkin, Donald, 179–185
taxol, nausea and vomiting, cannabis for
    management of, 141–144
Taylor, Bayard, 24

testosterone, cannabis impact on levels of,
    168–169
Thailand, cannabis consumption in,
    216–217
thandi, preparation of, 16–17
Thousand and One Nights, The (Arabian
    Nights), 19–20
Tibet, cannabis consumption in, 216
time
  alcohol effects on perceptions of, 99
  cannabis use and disorientation
    concerning, 86–94
tincture of cannabis
  preparation of, 16
  prohibitions against, 26
tobacco use
  cannabis consumption with, 207–209
  lung cancer and, 181–185
  marijuana smoke and, 175–185
Todd, Alexander, 33
tolerance development
  DSM-IV substance dependence criteria
    for, 107–108
  repeated cannabis use and, 105–113,
    167–168
toxicity of cannabis, 158–162
transporter, endocannabinoid biosynthesis,
    71–72
Treatise on Hemp, 13
TRPV-1 protein
  cardiovascular control and, 76
  endocannabinoid inactivation inhibition,
    78–79
  pain sensitivity, 75
Turner, William, 117

United Nations Single Convention on
    Narcotic Drugs, 232
United States
  anti-drug investigations in, 225–231
  arrest statistics for marijuana in,
    237–238
  cannabis cultivation in, 193–195
  cannabis prohibition in, 222–223

consuption patterns for cannabis in, 189–192
early use and subsequent prohibition of cannabis in, 25–26
history of hemp cultivation in, 23–25
medicinal use of cannabis in, 120–122
opposition to cannabis legalization in, 4–5, 21
rimonabant use in, 155
vaporization techniques, delta-9-tetrahydrocannabinol delivery through, 46–47
vascular system
cannabinoid effects on, 57–59
cannabis effects on, 164
Vietnam, cannabis consumption in, 216–217
visual sensitivity, cannabis intoxication and, 88–89
volatilization techniques, delta-9-tetrahydrocannabinol delivery through, 46–47

Walters, John, 12, 238
water pipes, for marijuana smoking, 15–16
Western medicine
cannabis in, 117–118
history of cannabis use in, 25
WIN55,212-2 compound
animal studies of effects of, 100–104
binding assays of, 52–54
development of, 38–39
neuroprotective effects of, 161–162
Wisset, Robert, 13
withdrawal syndrome, cannabis dependency and tolerance studies and, 110–113
Wood, H. C., 86–87
Wootton Report on cannabis use, 227–229
working memory, cannabis effects on, 97–98
World Health Organization (WHO)
cannabis use data from, 192
research on cannabis from, 231

Zion Coptic Church, 218–219

LaVergne, TN USA
26 May 2010
184044LV00002B/1/P

9 780195 328240